AN OUTLINE OF GERIATRICS
Second Edition

H. M. HODKINSON
M.A., D.M., F.R.C.P.

*Professor of Geriatric Medicine, Royal Postgraduate
Medical School, Hammersmith Hospital, London*

1981

ACADEMIC PRESS   London Toronto Sydney

GRUNE & STRATTON   New York San Francisco

ACADEMIC PRESS INC. (LONDON) LTD.
24/28 Oval Road,
London, NW1

United States Edition published by
GRUNE & STRATTON INC.
111 Fifth Avenue
New York, New York 10003

Copyright © 1981 by
ACADEMIC PRESS INC. (LONDON) LTD.
First edition published 1975

British Library Cataloguing in Publication Data
Hodkinson, H. M.
An outline of geriatrics.
1. Geriatrics
I. Title
618.97   RC952

ISBN (Academic Press) 0-12-792035-8
ISBN (Grune & Stratton) 0-8089-1397-2

LCCN 74-17996

PRINTED IN GREAT BRITAIN BY THE LAVENHAM PRESS LIMITED
LAVENHAM SUFFOLK

An Outline of Geriatrics

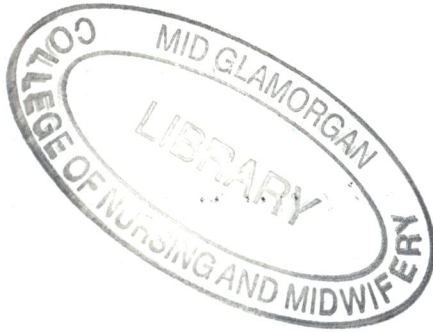

Preface to first edition

This short book is aimed particularly at interested medical students, especially those who choose geriatrics as the subject of an elective study period. However it is hoped that this intentionally brief account of the subject will also have a wider appeal. I hope it may prove useful to doctors in related fields and in General Practice who would like to advance their understanding of geriatrics without becoming embroiled in too detailed an account and that it similarly may be suitable to the requirements of nursing and rehabilitation staff who are concerned in the care of elderly.

To achieve the aim of a brief account of geriatrics which none the less conveys a coherent overall picture of the subject has involved considerable selection. I have tried to cover general aspects and principles reasonably fully but in dealing with diseases of the elderly have tried to keep very much to the most important examples. Many less common conditions thus find no mention. I have also tried to be sparing in my quotation of references, tending to confine these to the more accessible sources and to subjects of more topical interest or to recent reviews.

The book does not intend to serve as a reference work, for which purpose excellent books already exist. Rather it is hoped to provide an account which can be read completely without causing too much mental indigestion. It aims to complement larger reference works and perhaps to serve as a useful introduction to them.

London, September 1974   MALCOLM HODKINSON

Preface to second edition

This second edition of "An Outline of Geriatrics" closely follows the overall plan of the first. I have taken pains not to enlarge the book to any significant extent nor to change its essential characteristics whilst updating it. I have added suggestions for further reading at the ends of chapters but at the same time have reduced the number of references as well as revising them. I have given particular prominence to recent reviews and to the more readily accessible literature. Some omissions pointed out by helpful colleagues and reviewers have been remedied. As before the book aims to be a short and easily read introduction to geriatrics written from the standpoint of a practising physician in geriatric medicine.

London 1981   MALCOLM HODKINSON

Contents

1

What is Geriatrics?

Geriatrics is not a specialty which is easy to define. Unlike other specialities it does not deal with a circumscribed group of diseases, a system or a group of special techniques as do, for example, rheumatology, neurology or radiotherapy. Nor can it be clearly defined as dealing with a specific age group like paediatrics. For, although geriatrics is entirely concerned with the elderly, only a minority of the elderly admitted to hospital go to a department of geriatric medicine. This is inevitably so as the over 65 age-group accounts for roughly half of admissions to hospital. In practice, the 65-75 group is mainly dealt with by general departments and it is the elderly over 75 with whom the geriatrician is mostly concerned. We must therefore fall back on defining geriatrics in very general terms and quote the definition put forward by the British Geriatrics Society that

> Geriatrics is the branch of general medicine concerned with the clinical, preventive, remedial and social aspects of illness in the elderly.

HISTORICAL DEVELOPMENT OF GERIATRICS

Geriatrics in Great Britain effectively came into existence from the inception of the National Health Service in 1948 when the extensive reorganisation of medical services brought the problems of the elderly in hospital to proper notice. However the underlying changes which called for the emergence of geriatrics were of much longer duration. These were in the main the major changes in population structure, mortality patterns and morbidity which had occurred throughout the century. In 1901 there were 1.7 million people over 65 in Great Britain representing 5 per cent of the total population. Half a century later the proportion had risen to 11% and today exceeds 13%. These progressive rises in the proportions of higher age groups are shown in figure 1. They have resulted almost entirely from falling mortality rates in childhood and middle life, due principally to prevention and effective treatment of infections, and not to any significant gain in longevity in old age. Thus in the first half of this century death rates (for females) fell by 87 per cent for children under 15, by 74 per cent for the 15-44 age-group and by 56 per cent for those aged 45-65. In striking contrast to this, mortality for females over 65 fell by only 2 per cent.

The old make disproportionately high demands on hospital services so that their progressive proportional increase, which is expected to continue for some years to come, means that the hospital service has had to adapt to the

1

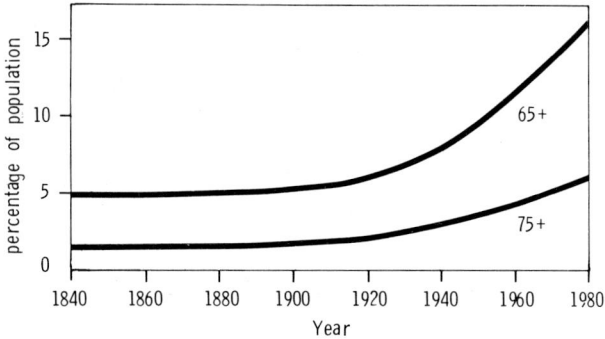

Fig. 1. Increases in the percentage of elderly persons in the population of Great Britain. The relatively greater increase in the over 75s is shown.

different problems posed by elderly patients who have come to occupy some two-thirds of the total beds.

The increase in numbers of the elderly provided the basis for the development of geriatrics but the early stages of that development were shaped by unfortunate influences from the past. In former times the Poor Law had thrown the destitute haphazardly together whether their problem was poverty, physical or mental illness or disability. Under this enduring system, two distinct kinds of hospital had developed; the voluntary hospitals and the Poor Law institutions or workhouses. The false assumption that there were two corresponding categories of patients, the acute patients and the chronic patients, arose from this dichotomy. The new National Health Service inherited these old attitudes as well as the old buildings. McKeown (1960) has summarised these prejudices:

> Acute work was conceived as something effective from the patient's point of view and interesting from the point of view of the doctor; being of short duration it could be financed by voluntary funds or by private contract between doctor and patient. Chronic work, in contrast, was unlikely to be effective, was unrewarding for doctor and nurse and, because of its association with destitution, had to be provided at public expense.

The two-tier system resulted in two very different standards of care and it was the "acute" hospitals which achieved the higher standards and the greater prestige and were responsible for the training of doctors and nurses. This led to those who were trained lacking knowledge and interest in the problems of the elderly, the chronically sick or disabled and the mentally ill.

When administrative unification took place at the onset of the National Health Service, the poor standards of work with these groups of people could no longer be overlooked and efforts to bring back these neglected areas into the main stream of medical care could properly begin.

In the case of the care of the elderly, an earlier lead had been given by pioneers such as Marjory Warren and Trevor Howell who had shown that the application of proper diagnostic and therapeutic measures to the elderly hospital patient was capable of giving good results, far beyond the expectations of that time. Geriatric departments began to be set up, taking over responsibility for the former "chronic wards". These first departments were able to confirm and develop the effectiveness of the new geriatric approach to the hospital treatment of the elderly. The new specialty slowly gained acceptance because of the results it achieved and is now fully established as a major branch of medicine with departments throughout the country.

THE GERIATRIC DEPARTMENT

What geriatrics is can perhaps be best explained by looking at the work and aims of a geriatric department.

The Patients

The patients are most obviously characterised by their age, which on average is around 80 for most departments. Commonly, though there is a lower age limit of 65 for admission, there is quite heavy selection of patients on the basis of a poor prognosis, multiple disease, social pathology, confusion, incontinence or immobility. This selection is likely to be particularly marked among the younger elderly (65-75) of whom only a minority are admitted to the geriatric department in most districts. In contrast the over 75s are relatively unselected, the majority going to the geriatric service. However, a few geriatric departments cater for virtually all hospital medical admissions for those over 65 in their district.

So in most districts, whilst in the population some two-thirds of the over 65 age-group are under 75, this 65-75 group may only provide a third of the admissions to a geriatric department. Figure 2 shows the age distribution of

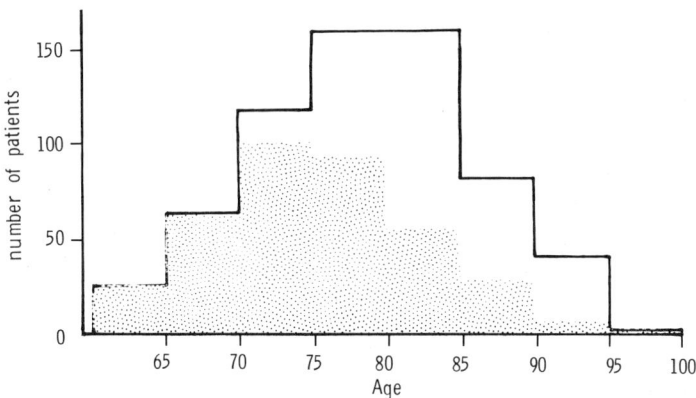

Fig. 2. Age distribution for 1023 consecutive patients admitted to the geriatric department of Hammersmith Hospital (males as shaded histogram, females unshaded). Average age was 78 for men and 81 for women and there was a marked female preponderance in the higher age groups, women comprising 64% of admissions overall.

admissions to my own department as a typical example but also illustrates the stiking preponderance of females who typically provide about two-thirds of a department's admissions.

Apart from this excess of females, there is also over-representation of the single, widowed and lower social classes.

Patients are admitted from a defined catchment area. This arrangement, which is shared by only a small number of other services such as psychiatry, maternity and chest diseases, reflects the common need for strong local social links for the service to be fully effective. The geriatric catchment area reduces freedom of choice by patients and referring doctors but does ensure that "the buck stops here", an important safeguard in an area where there is heavy pressure on resources and there are all too often waiting lists for admission.

Medical Conditions

The medical conditions which favour selection of patients for geriatric admission are, particularly, multiple disease, illness in the setting of pre-existing physical or mental disability and physical illness accompanied by mental disturbance. Elderly patients are more likely to be referred if they have social disabilities or if the need for lengthy hospital stay or terminal care is foreseen. Patients who have a major rehabilitation requirement, for example those with stroke, Parkinsonism or locomotor disease, are more likely to be selected.

Special Facilities and Attributes

Special facilities and attributes of a geriatric department consist first of all in a commitment to the care of the elderly and interest in their problems. Medical staff will have special experience and knowledge of disease in the elderly, particularly the problems of multiple disease, psychiatric and psychological factors and rehabilitational and social implications. There will be special skill in the management of discharges and arrangements for further care in the community and close links will be maintained with local services for the elderly. There will be appropriate rehabilitation facilities and usually some system of progressive patient care to assist the provision of the most suitable care for the individual patient throughout the stages of his hospital stay. Nursing will be specially geared to the needs of the elderly with particular skill in managing frail, confused, incontinent and immobile patients and in the prevention of pressure sores and avoidance of unnecessary dependency and institutionalisation.

Function and Aims of a Geriatric Department

The function and aims of a geriatric department can be summarised as the provision of an effective and comprehensive hospital service for the elderly which fully caters for their investigation, treatment and rehabilitation and has their return to the community as the expected outcome. Terminal care, long-stay care of irremediable patients and social admissions such as "holiday admissions" will also be an integral part of the service although accounting for only a minority of the patients who are admitted. The department aims to provide the best standards of medical and nursing care for the elderly, whether their illness might be termed "acute" or "chronic". In addition departments seek to improve and develop hospital and community care of the elderly and to be active in the appropriate research and teaching activities.

Psychogeriatrics

In much the same way that geriatric medicine evolved within the field of internal medicine, so in more recent years there has been a parallel development of psychogeriatrics within psychiatry. However, though practically all health districts now have a geriatric service, only a minority have a specialist psychogeriatric service and the remainder still look to general psychiatrist for the care of the elderly.

Pioneer psychogeriatric departments, dealing with the full range of psychiatric illness in old age, not just with dementia, have clearly shown the benefits of replacing old custodial patterns of care with more active approaches. The value of close liaison between the psychogeriatric and geriatric services with the setting up of joint assessment facilities is also of proven value.

Further Reading

Evans, J G (1978) Demography and resources, Medicine (series 3) *I*, 12-14.

Hall, M R P (1978) Requirement and utilisation of resources by the elderly, p 155-164 in Recent advances in geriatric medicine, Ed. Isaacs, B, Churchill Livingstone, Edinburgh.

Silver, C P (1978) Patterns of delivery of care by departments of geriatric medicine, p 121-130, in Recent advances in geriatric medicine, Ed. Isaacs, B, Churchill Livingstone, Edinburgh.

2

How Elderly Patients are Different

Elderly patients differ in many ways from the young, indeed such distinctions underlie the separate existence of Geriatrics as a medical specialty. We see these differences in the type and number of the diseases affecting the elderly patient, in his reactions to disease and in the special features of the elderly person as a patient.

DISEASE IN THE ELDERLY

Multiple Pathology

A striking feature of disease in the elderly is that it is very commonly multiple. This occurence of multiple pathology calls for considerable re-orientation of thinking as classical medical teaching, mainly based on experience of illness in earlier age-groups, has always stressed the importance of unifying all the findings of history, examination and investigation into the framework of a single diagnosis. This approach is often untenable in geriatric work where multiple diagnoses are the rule and a single diagnosis exceptional. So, whilst we must not overlook a unifying diagnosis where this is appropriate, far more often we need to make multiple diagnoses and may find very different clinical pictures because of the interaction of different pathologies. These differences and the greater complexities of treatment in the setting of multiple disease will be considered further in later chapters. The multiplicity of disease in the old is partly accounted for by the accumulation of non-lethal diseases which are often degenerative in character, for example osteoarthritis, osteoporosis, cataract, deafness and varicose veins. Other more dangerous degenerative conditions become more common with rise in age, for example atherosclerosis, the dementias and emphysema. Cancer, pernicious anaemia, thyrotoxicosis and myxoedema are all more prevalent, perhaps because of deterioration of immune mechanisms. Obesity, diabetes, depression and many other diseases also occur more frequently in the old.

"Missing" Diseases

Other diseases become less common in older age-groups for reasons which are not always apparent, for example infective hepatitis or acute glomerulonephritis are practically never seen in advanced old age. Some diseases of a highly lethal nature and whose incidence rises with age are paradoxically uncommon in the very aged, perhaps because susceptible individuals are eliminated at earlier ages, thus severe hypertension or severe bronchitis are not often encountered in patients over eighty.

Differential Diagnosis

Because of these factors differential diagnosis is considerably modified in old age. Thus senile or arteriosclerotic dementia are the likely causes of progressive dementia in an old person while the differential diagnosis in a middle-aged patient would be very different and such conditions as space occupying lesion, Alzheimer's disease and Huntington's chorea would be relatively greater in importance.

ALTERED REACTIONS TO DISEASE

The elderly react very differently to disease processes and these modifications are sufficient to require full discussion in later chapters. There are differences in presentation of illness, for example due to alteration of pain mechanisms and temperature response. Mental disturbance is far more likely to occur as a response to physical illness and rehabilitation is far more often necessary because of the increased tendency for general deterioration to occur during periods of illness and the consequent enforced inactivity.

It is these differences, rather than any poorer capacity to respond to appropriate treatment for the underlying disease, which underlie the less favourable outcome of illness in the old and the higher mortalities which are encountered.

THE ELDERLY PERSON AND HIS BACKGROUND

The elderly patient is old as well as ill. Prior to his illness he had many disadvantages. Old age may bring with it some memory impairment. Mobility often deteriorates because of osteoarthritis, neurological disabilities or even due to such homely conditions as painful feet from corns or bunions. Poorer mobility coupled with deteriorating mechanisms of postural control makes old people more vulnerable to falls and other accidents and these are more likely to result in fracture because of the high prevalence of osteoporosis. Visual impairment and deafness are major problems for many old people. Changes in bladder function with age mean that incontinence far more readily results from extra stresses, for example from urinary infection or the use of a diuretic drug. Finally, a general slowing down and increasing frailty are often found in advanced old age. The aged person may still be able to carry out accustomed activities such as dressing but takes far longer and needs to make a much bigger effort than before. The young need to be patient and sympathetic when meeting this situation.

The elderly often lack a role in our present day work-oriented society and are financially at a disadvantage in comparison with the young. In consequence they often live in old and inconvenient housing with poor facilities. They may have difficulties in affording sufficient heating and may be obliged to adopt an unsuitable diet too heavily dependent on cheap foods such as bread. The combination of poverty, disability, lack of status and lack of being valued by others leads to poor morale with restriction of interests in many old people and perhaps underlies the high frequency of depression in the age group.

Under-reporting of Illness

The elderly can be forgiven for taking a somewhat pessimistic view of what life in general and medicine in particular have to offer. This is summed up by the phrase one so often hears when talking to an old patient, "well, what can you expect at my age". The consequence is that the elderly often fail to seek necessary help and advice and the under-reporting of illness and disability presents a major challenge to medical and social services for the elderly. Dementia, depression, locomotor diseases, urinary tract disorders, failing vision and deafness are particularly commonly unreported.

Need for Social Support

Because of their physical, mental and social disabilities, the old often need the support of other people to carry on their lives in the community. Families supply a great amount of such support but are too often accused of neglecting their old relatives despite the findings of objective studies which have shown that rejection of the elderly by their families is altogether exceptional. Often the caring relatives are elderly themselves: if the patient is 95, the daughter caring for her may be well within the geriatric age-group!

Lack of family support is more often due to lack of family and the superior survival of the elderly female makes her especially vulnerable in this respect as she commonly survives her husband and not rarely her other close relatives. Children may be too far away to help, a penalty of modern social mobility. In the absence of family, neighbours, home-helps, "meals on wheels" and the district nurse can play a vital role.

Bereavement or illness of a helper can strike a severe blow to the ill or disabled old person both in terms of the loss of physical help and its effect on morale.

CONCLUSIONS

The elderly patient is characterised by the multiplicity of his diseases and the background of pre-existing disability. Psychiatric disturbance commonly accompanies physical disease and illness occurs in the setting of social disabilities and hardship. The old often fail to report their illness or disability and to seek proper help and assessment of their illness calls for the consideration of activity and medical, psychiatric and social factors.

Further Reading

Anderson, Sir Ferguson (1978) The early detection and prevention of disease in the elderly, p. 143-153, in Recent advances in geriatric medicine, Ed. Isaacs, B, Churchill Livingstone, Edinburgh.

Brearley, C P (1975) Social work, ageing and society, Routledge & Kegan Paul, London

Simpson, R G (1974) Disease patterns in the elderly, British Journal of Hospital Medicine, *12*, 660-677.

3

The History

History taking in the elderly patient presents many special features and difficulties in comparison with younger adults.

MENTAL CONFUSION

Confused patients present obvious difficulties. However some demented patients can keep up a misleadingly effective conversational facade so that much time may be taken up with the history before it becomes apparent that the patient's account is quite unreliable because of its internal inconsistencies. Because of such instances, the administration of some brief form of routine mental test (Hodkinson, 1972) can be useful in alerting the doctor. However, if care is taken, quite severely demented patients may be capable of giving a history that is of value, although this will need to be carefully cross-checked by interviewing relatives or neighbours. The inexperienced are more often likely to give up too readily and the note "history unobtainable, patient confused" is seen more often than it should be.

DEAFNESS

The common occurrence of deafness in the elderly is another major barrier in history taking. One danger resulting from this is that the doctor tends to assume that all old patients are deaf and falls into the error of speaking loudly in every case. His elderly patients with normal hearing may be very offended by this and some may point this out with some heat! It is not easy to re-establish good rapport after having been justifiably put in one's place in this way.

When the patient is recognised as being deaf, it is more helpful to speak slowly and clearly and in a position where one's face is clearly visible so as to give an opportunity for lip reading. The extra information from lip reading, even in those who are not particularly expert, may make a great contribution to their understanding of what is partially heard. Furthermore the eye contact which results from face to face conversation is an important factor in maintaining the patient's attention and concentration.

It is important that a patient with a hearing aid is encouraged to use it and the ill person may need help to fix and regulate it. Very deaf patients without aids may call for other measures. An ear trumpet or the doctor's own

stethoscope as a makeshift substitute may be helpful. Occasionally a special
amplifier and headphones may be of assistance when other aids are
ineffective (Hall, 1973). When these methods fail pencil and paper can be
used; although history taking in this way is slow it is worth while to persevere.
Not bothering to make the effort to communicate is likely to be very
demoralising to the deaf patient.

Few of the elderly deaf have knowledge of sign language so that it is not a
useful skill for the doctor to acquire, however the potential usefulness of
ordinary gesture is not to be ignored.

CONCENTRATION

Concentration is often poor in the elderly patient who is frail or confused and
fatigue and inattention may develop after a very short time. When this is so,
the doctor should aim to break up history taking into a number of short
sessions. Often the day of admission is not the best time for history taking
because it has been an exhausting day for the ill patient and one may do
better to leave history taking until the following day, except for its broadest
outlines. Dyspnoea is a particular difficulty and detailed history taking may
have to wait until some improvement has resulted from initial treatment.

COOPERATION

Cooperation of the elderly patient is often less than ideal. Time invested in
the establishment of good rapport is unlikely to be wasted. It helps if the
doctor appears unhurried and is prepared to pass the time of day for a little
while before plunging into the detailed history. Physical contact can be a
help, holding the hand of the nervous old patient, a reassuring hand on the
shoulder or the more formal handshake can all help the patient to feel more
at ease. The essential is to convey interest in the patient as a person in his
own right.

Despite the best of approaches, patients may be unforthcoming, apprehensive, evasive or aggressive. Depressed patients are particularly likely to be unforthcoming because of their apathy and feelings of hopelessness. Confused
patients may deny illness or may react to the frustration of questions which
overtax their defective memory by aggression and such remarks as "why do
you keep asking me all these stupid questions, go and ask somebody else".

IDIOSYNCRASIES

Many old people are rambling historians and when this is coupled with some
degree of memory impairment history taking becomes a very diffuse and
laborious process unless the interviewing doctor can learn how to direct and
curb the old person without offence. One has to make use of many more

leading questions than is usual in taking a history from younger patients and may have to use them to draw the old person back from some digression. Problems arise because the old are often more imprecise in their account, particularly with regard to duration and chronology but also in such areas as the description of pain or its localisation. A danger of using direct questioning too extensively is that the old are particularly likely to agree too readily to whatever the question suggests out of a misguided wish to please the questioner.

The elderly, understandably, tend to have "old fashioned" views of medicine so that what they think important may differ greatly from the doctor's assessment. A striking example is that of their reverence for "the bowels", the functioning of which is likely to be described in obsessional detail.

Confusion may also arise because of the different use of language by the old. "Giddiness", for example, which in the young can often be equated with vertigo, seldom indicates this in an old person but is more often used to describe feelings of insecurity, unsteadiness, fear of falling or faintness. Differences in expectations may also lead to significant symptoms being discounted by the old person who regards them as "normal for my age". Breathlessness, rheumatic pains, deteriorating mobility or memory failure are commonly disregarded in this way.

CORROBORATION OF THE HISTORY

Because of the difficulties of history taking in elderly patients, it is often necessary to check the story with relatives or friends. Where, because of severe illness or obvious confusion, gross difficulty in history taking can be foreseen, it is often useful to do this in advance of interviewing the patient; in such circumstances the general practitioner's referring letter can be of inestimable value. It is better that such checking of the history is not done with the patient present as it can lead to unpleasant disagreements and also may be unhelpful to the patient's morale if it becomes clear that his account is thought to be unreliable or of subordinate importance.

DIFFERENCES OF EMPHASIS

Much of history taking in the old is closely similar to that in middle life but there are some differences of emphasis. Some aspects are of less importance in the old, for example family history and occupational history are less often relevant but should not however be ignored. Other areas are of greater importance and the major examples are discussed below. Further instances are the special senses, locomotor system, diet and the occurrence of falls or "queer turns".

ASSESSMENT OF ACTIVITY

The levels of mobility and everyday activities are of considerable interest as deterioration in them may be an important indication of physical or mental disease having developed. Furthermore, the previous levels of mobility and activity need to be known if realistic aims and plans for rehabilitation and discharge are to be made. As well as the ability to walk, it is useful to enquire into ability to climb stairs, whether the patient is housebound, what household duties are performed and whether there are any problems regarding continence.

SOCIAL HISTORY

The social circumstances of the old person are often central to effective planning of his treatment and care. One needs to know what social support the patient has had and may expect in the future and what social pressures or changes may have affected his health and capacity for independence. Special areas of concern are housing, finance, family support, isolation, support from social services and the nature of the patient's personal relationships with those supporting him. In taking the social history one may gain valuable insight into the patient's personality, motivation and future plans.

MENTAL HEALTH

The psychiatric aspects of history taking will be more fully considered in a later chapter. The main concerns are in the recognition of depression and of dementia and confusional states, all of which are common in the elderly.

DRUG HISTORY

An accurate and detailed knowledge of drugs being taken is of particular importance in the elderly who are especially vulnerable to side effects. In addition, the elderly not infrequently fail to take medicines which have been prescribed. Sometimes one wonders if they are not guided in this by a useful instinct of self preservation as, regretably, over-prescribing is all too common. However, neglect to continue to take such key maintenance treatments as thyroxine for myxoedema or digitalis and diuretics for cardiac failure and the consequent relapse are unfortunately common causes of illness and of hospital admission in the elderly.

CONCLUSIONS

Practice, skill and experience are needed in order to obtain adequate histories in geriatric work. However, as is the case in younger age-groups, a good history is essential to proper diagnosis and treatment. The time and effort involved in obtaining an adequate history represent a vital investment and attempts to take short-cuts with the history taking are unwise and potentially dangerous.

Further Reading

Caird, F I & Judge, T G (1979) Assessment of the elderly patient, 2nd edition, Pitman Medical, London.

4

The Physical Examination

The physical examination of the elderly patient needs to be comprehensive and thorough. In general, physical examination is closely similar to that in the young but, as with history taking, there are some areas of difficulty and others with special importance and it is these areas which will be the subject of this chapter.

COOPERATION

As is the case with history taking, poor cooperation may cause problems during physical examination. Deafness, confusion, frailty, fatigue and poor concentration may be factors. Dyspnoea, pain or weakness are added difficulties. Immobility and physical helplessness mean that much more assistance is required during examination. When the elderly are to be examined at home this need for physical assistance is coupled with the problem of excessive clothing. Even on the hottest summer day one finds elderly patients enshrouded in innumerable layers of clothing and removal of these is a time consuming process which can be taxing both in terms of physical assistance and of persuasion! General practitioners or geriatricians who must examine the elderly in their own homes unassisted need to have cultivated the special skills of undressing and positioning overclad and immobile old people and must resist the temptation to give up the attempt to carry out an adequate physical examination.

GENERAL ASPECTS OF EXAMINATION

In the general part of the examination of the elderly patient one may get useful diagnostic leads from general appearance. The characteristic facies and voice changes of myxoedema, the pallor of anaemia, the sallow pigmentation of sub-acute bacterial endocarditis or the peaches and cream appearance of pernicious anaemia are examples. The patient's general demeanour may suggest depression or hyperkinetic behaviour may indicate thyrotoxicosis.

Dehydration is an important finding but signs of skin inelasticity are less helpful because the skin of the arms, neck or body is normally rather inelastic in the old. Turgor can more reliably be assessed using a fold of the lateral part of the cheek. A dry tongue is an important indicator of dehydration but may be due simply to mouth breathing.

Examination of the mouth often shows angular stomatitis but this is commonly due to poorly fitting dentures or edentulousness rather than deficiency. Atrophic glossitis may indicate pernicious anaemia or carious fangs alert one to the possibility of sub-acute bacterial endocarditis.

It is important to examine the breasts as a routine as cancer of the breast is not uncommon. Sometimes very advanced breast cancers are found at a routine examination in elderly women who, guessing the correct diagnosis but fearing surgical treatment, have deliberately avoided seeking medical advice.

In winter months particularly the possibility of hypothermia needs to be remembered; an abdomen that feels cool to the examining hand can be a useful pointer and should lead to the measurement of rectal temperature using a low reading thermometer.

CARDIOVASCULAR SYSTEM

The blood pressure is frequently found to be elevated at the initial examination of an old person but repeated determinations on succeeding days most often show a return to acceptable levels. The pulse is irregular in many old people, most often due to auricular fibrillation although there are many other possibilities. Routine electrocardiography is valuable both in the diagnosis of arrhythmias and also because of the frequency of ischaemic heart disease and of clinically silent infarction.

The heart may be clinically enlarged and murmurs are common. Most often heard are aortic systolic and mitral systolic murmurs but faint aortic diastolic murmurs are to be heard quite often by an experienced observer and usually indicate mild aortic incompetence due to aortic dilatation. Mitral stenosis is occasional and not usually severe.

Congestive cardiac failure is common but care needs to be taken that it is not overdiagnosed by mistakenly regarding mechanical leg oedema in immobile or arthritic patients as being cardiac in origin.

Peripheral vascular disease is frequent, although often asymptomatic, so that it is sound clinical practice to examine the peripheral pulses of the legs and to look for evidence of skin ischaemia as a routine.

ALIMENTARY SYSTEM

Examination of the abdomen may be hampered by the old person's inability to relax the abdominal musculature and if one then asks him to relax the most usual result is board-like rigidity of the abdominal wall! Aneurismal dilatation of the abdominal aorta is not rare but the normal sized aorta can often be palpated easily in thin old people. It is important not to confuse the palpable aorta with other abdominal masses. This applies to the scybala that are so commonly palpable in the descending colon or elsewhere in the abdomen. An established transverse abdominal skin crease can be a useful indication of old vertebral collapse, typically due to osteoporosis.

Rectal examination must never be omitted in examining the elderly patient. Faecal impaction is an important cause of discomfort or of spurious diarrhoea while benign prostatic hypertrophy, carcinoma of the prostate and rectal carcinoma are all far from rare.

RESPIRATORY SYSTEM

Kyphosis and scoliosis can interfere with examination of the chest and many old patients have difficulty in taking adequate deep breaths. Old pleural thickening or pulmonary fibrosis may be present or there may be some degree of emphysema. All these factors increase the difficulties of the diagnosis of chest pathology from physical signs in the elderly. Another snag is that basal crepitations may be heard when no lung pathology is present. In view of these facts, routine chest radiography is strongly advisable in the ill old person.

CENTRAL NERVOUS SYSTEM

Central nervous system disease is common in old age but unfortunately examination of this system is particularly likely to overtax the cooperation and endurance of old patients. This particularly applies to sensory testing where the rapid fatigue of concentration can easily lead to misleading results of the examination.

The significance of some central nervous system signs in the old is open to debate (Prakash and Stern, 1973). In particular, small muscle wasting in the hands is seldom of neurological significance and probably related to arthritis and disuse. Tendon reflexes, especially the ankle jerks, may be lost and so may vibration sense in the legs and these abnormalities probably do not as a rule indicate neurological disease.

Because of difficulties in relaxation, tone can be difficult to assess. In such cases the recognition of Parkinsonism can be problematical as the glabella sign is of little diagnostic value in the aged, and many false positives occur. The head drop test (Wartenberg, 1952) can then be useful. The patient is examined lying flat on the back without a pillow. The examiners hand is placed beneath the occiput and, when the patient has relaxed, the head is thrown up suddenly and allowed to fall back. Normally the head falls back hard onto the examiner's hand but if there is Parkinsonian rigidity, its descent is slowed and in the more severe cases may not occur at all so as to leave the head suspended above the bed, the "psychic pillow" sign.

LOCOMOTOR SYSTEM

Examination of the locomotor system and the general assessment of mobility and gait is particularly relevant in old age. A small pace gait is often seen in the absence of neurological causes such as Parkinsonism. Difficulties in balance need to be noted and may be due to mechanical causes such as lateral instability of the knees or to central nervous system conditions.

The joints should be systematically examined and osteoarthritis, which is a usual finding, should be assessed as to severity and extent. Rheumatoid arthritis, usually old and inactive clinically, is not uncommon particularly in females but may be mistakenly diagnosed when osteoarthritis of the hands is accompanied by Bouchard's nodes of the proximal interphalangeal joints so as to superficially mimic rheumatoid changes. Joint effusions need to be looked for, traumatic effusions into osteoarthritis knees being a common possibility.

The occurrence of fractures needs to be remembered, fracture of the femoral neck is often overlooked in the arthritic old person who has had many falls. Vertebral collapse may show itself by local deformity or tenderness as well as by the transverse abdominal crease already referred to. Sacro-iliac tenderness is another important cause of low back pain.

The feet should be fully examined as painful corns and calluses, neglected toe nails and onychogryphoses or ischemic ulceration can all result in impaired mobility.

URO-GENITAL SYSTEM

Urinary retention, which may be chronic and with overflow and not associated with abdominal pain or discomfort, is an important finding and the distended bladder must not be overlooked during abdominal examination.

In the elderly female, the "lost" ring is worthy of note. A ring pessary may have been fitted many years before and completely forgotten only to be rediscovered on rectal or vaginal examination. My "personal best" was the finding of a ring that had been lost for forty-three years! Amazingly it has only resulted in some vaginal discharge in recent months but its removal involved piecemeal extraction of the deeply embedded ring.

THE EYES

An assessment of vision needs to be made and the commonest cause for impairment of vision is cataract. The pupils are not infrequently irregular due to degenerative rather than neurological disease. The pupils are often small so that adequate examination of the fundi may call for dilatation using a short acting mydriatic.

Fundoscopy most often reveals arteriosclerotic vascular changes, sometimes diabetic retinitis but many other pathologies may be encountered from time to time. With dilatation of the pupils, most fundi can be adequately visualised despite pupillary abnormalities or cataracts (other than the very severe ones) and this potentially valuable part of the examination of the old person should not be unnecessarily omitted.

THE EARS

Deafness is common and needs to be assessed. Wax in the ears is a common and treatable cause so that auriscopy is an indispensable part of the examination of the old person who is hard of hearing.

THE SKIN

Common findings include senile (seborrhoeic) warts, senile purpura and scars of old varicose ulcers or of herpes zoster but these are of no great practical significance. Rodent ulcers are particularly common in old age and are most often seen on the face especially on the eyelids, near the inner canthus or behind the ear. Intertrigo is a common finding in the obese, occuring under the breasts and in the groins. Dupuytren's contracture may be seen, particularly in old men. Pruritus is sometimes a troublesome symptom in the old and scabies should be remembered as a possible cause. One should look for the characteristic burrows between the fingers and in the flexures of the wrists and elbows.

Further Reading

Caird, F I & Judge, T G (1979) Assessment of the elderly patient, 2nd edition, Pitman Medical, London.
Wright, W B (1977) How to examine an old person, Lancet *1*. 1145-6.

5

Investigation of the Elderly

POLICY

As a group, elderly patients have tended to have been under-investigated in the past on the basis that accurate diagnosis was unnecessary as nothing useful could be achieved at their age. Geriatric experience has shown this view to be totally inappropriate and that much treatable disease can be found among elderly patients who are comprehensively investigated. Clearly, excessive investigational zeal is to be avoided and the likelihood of benefit to the patient must outweigh the unpleasantness or danger of any investigational procedures. Also investigation for purely "academic" interest is to be avoided, for example bronchoscopy to confirm carcinoma of the bronchus when there is no intention to undertake further treatment in view of the patient's general condition. Such reservations, which in any case apply to all age groups, should not be exaggerated and used to rationalise and excuse the tendency for the elderly to be denied the benefits of thorough investigation.

INTERPRETATION

A problem which commonly arises in investigating the elderly is to decide what is normal and what is abnormal. Are the standards the same as for the young or can some departure from the usual standards be accepted as due to age? Many such questions are yet to be fully answered and this applies particularly to laboratory tests where the "normal ranges" have usually been assessed in volunteers who are all young. Often highly selected groups such as students or technicians have been used so that very young males predominate. Better balanced groups have commonly been blood donors but this involves a maximum age of 65. The usual textbook "normal ranges" cannot therefore be applied automatically to the old. When multiple tests are applied to an elderly patient, several may be somewhat outside the conventional "normal ranges" and considerable judgement is then required to decide which departures are likely to be relevant and call for further investigation.

RADIOLOGICAL INVESTIGATION

A chest X-ray should be part of the routine investigation of all ill old people. This is because of the special difficulties of physical examination of the chest in the old already mentioned in Chapter 4 so that chest disease cannot be excluded on the basis of absence of findings. The routine chest film in practice yields a heavy crop of abnormalities.

Some changes are associated with age and of no clinical significance, for example calcification of the costal cartilages, bronchial rings, larynx and hyoid are common with increasing age. Aortic calcification and unfolding is very frequent. Kyphosis and scoliosis are common and add to difficulties of interpretation, especially of heart size. Paget's disease may be picked up from the chest film; clavicle, head of the humerus and the coracoid process being the common sites. Bone metastases, usually from breast or prostate, must not be overlooked.

In the lungs, pneumonia is a common finding even in those with no physical signs. Primary and secondary carcinoma, tuberculosis, pulmonary fibrosis, pulmonary oedema, effusion and pulmonary embolism are all far from rare.

Because of their frailty and immobility, radiography can be taxing in the elderly both to the patient and the staff of the radiology department. This needs to be fully considered when embarking on more major X-ray procedures such as barium studies, I.V.P. or arteriography. It has been shown that whilst barium meal often gives clinically useful information, the more taxing barium enema is frequently unrewarding. Arteriography carries considerable risks in arteriosclerotic old patients and should only be performed for compelling reasons and where treatment will be practicable if there are significant findings.

Some radiological abnormalities are so commonly present but symptomless in old age, that their demonstration is of little value in deciding whether symptoms can be attributed to the abnormality. Examples here are diverticula of the colon and cervical spondylitic changes.

Constipation can present radiological problems. Despite intensive and protracted efforts in preparing the patient for radiography, faecal masses may make it impossible to obtain satisfactory views for I.V.P. or barium enema and on occasions one may have to give up gracefully!

HAEMATOLOGICAL INVESTIGATION

The normal values for haemoglobin, the packed cell volume, mean corpuscular volume and other indices, platelets, prothrombin time and other coagulation tests are unchanged in old age. Anaemia (haemoglobin below 12 g/dl) is sufficiently common to warrant routine haemoglobin and blood count in all ill old people. The mean corpuscular volume (M.C.V.) as determined by modern electronic counting machines such as the "Coulter S" is a powerful tool in the separation of the two common types of anaemia, iron deficiency and megaloblastic. A raised M.C.V. is a better screening test for megaloblastic anaemia than the more difficult and fallible serum B_{12} and red cell folate estimations. Most elderly patients tolerate marrow puncture well when this is necessary for the confirmation of haematological diagnosis and this investigation need not be omitted simply on the grounds of age. Marrow iron stores are a better guide to iron status than iron binding saturation which may give misleading results in ill old people. In the diagnosis of megaloblastic anaemia the red cell folate is a far more reliable guide as to folate status than the serum folate whilst B_{12} absorption tests with and without intrinsic factor can confirm the diagnosis of pernicious anaemia without the need to subject the old person to gastric intubation to demonstrate achlorhydria.

The white cell count is less often helpful than in the young as leucocytosis in response to infection is less often seen. The range for the white cell count is in fact lower in old age, 3000-9000 compared to 4000-12,000 for the young.

BIOCHEMICAL INVESTIGATION

The difficulties of defining "normal ranges" apply particularly to the biochemical investigation of the old. For some parameters, ranges un-doubtedly rise with age and can be shown to rise even in middle life (Roberts, 1967; Keating et al., 1969). Thus the values for urea rise with age but, while accepting somewhat higher urea levels as "normal" for an older person, it seems clear that these do indicate poorer renal function which is a factor of significance whether one regards the deterioration as due to ageing or disease. The rise for urea is paralleled by rises in creatinine and uric acid. In contrast, albumin shows a fall with age. Other parameters show differences in old age but the significance of these is obscured by the possibility of disturbance by unrecognised disease. Alkaline phosphatase is an example here; studies of apparently healthy old people show a higher range in old age but this finding is probably due to inclusion of unrecognised cases of Paget's disease and osteomalacia. Some biochemical parameters appear to have ranges which are unchanged from those in earlier age-groups and these include sodium, potassium, chloride and bicarbonate (Leask et al., 1973).

When biochemical tests are applied to ill old people, interpretation is further complicated by the effects of therapy and of interaction of disease processes (Hodkinson, 1977). Particularly frequent are the effects of impaired renal function and of altered serum proteins. Altered renal function may be responsible for elevation of uric acid, creatinine and phosphate as well as urea but may also alter electrolytes and calcium. Changes in serum proteins affect levels of substances that are substantially bound to proteins in the blood such as calcium (bound to albumin), thyroid hormone (mainly bound to a specific carrier protein, thyroxine-binding-globulin) and serum iron (bound to a specific carrier protein also). All these carrier proteins tend to fall to lower levels in ill old people so that the measured level of calcium, thyroxine or iron will appear abnormally low. An

---

NORMAL RANGES UNCHANGED IN OLD AGE
serum sodium, serum potassium, serum chloride, serum bicarbonate, S.G.O.T., bilirubin, acid phosphatase, serum T4

NORMAL RANGES RAISED IN OLD AGE
alkaline phosphatase, globulin, urea, creatinine, uric acid, calcium (in women), E.S.R.

NORMAL RANGES DECREASED IN OLD AGE
albumin, phosphate (in men), serum T3, serum iron, T.I.B.C., W.B.C.

---

example of the effects of therapy is the occurrence of hyponatraemia or hypokalaemia with diuretic therapy due to increased renal loss of sodium and potassium. More complex effects include those of the sex and anabolic steroids which may produce abnormal thyroid function tests by altering thyroxine-binding-globulin as well as lowered calcium and phosphorus levels.

Despite difficulties in interpretation, routine screening of ill elderly patients for common treatable diseases is of established value. Particularly worthwhile is screening for osteomalacia, thyroid disease and diabetes, all with diagnosis rates of 2-5 per cent. Biochemical screening tests on geriatric patients thus usefully include calcium, phosphorus, alkaline phosphatase, albumin, serum T4 and T3-uptake or TSH, random blood sugar, urea and electrolytes. Questions as to the value of similar routine screening in apparently healthy old people are yet to be adequately answered. Certainly it would be unwise to assume that the yields would be in any way comparable to those in ill old people.

ELECTROCARDIOGRAPHY

The E.C.G. is a worthwhile routine examination as arrhythmias, ischaemia and infarction are so frequent in ill old people. This is particularly so as infarction is so often not accompanied by pain and may present in a very non-specific way. Few hospital geriatric patients have completely normal E.C.Gs, and the investigation can often give highly relevant information.

ELECTROENCEPHALOGRAPHY

Electroencephalography has a small but useful role in demonstrating focal cerebral disorder but more especially in the recognition of epilepsy as the cause of episodes of transient loss of consciousness.

URINALYSIS

Urine testing for sugar is of importance because diabetes is common but the absence of glycosuria may mislead because many elderly diabetics also have a high renal threshold for sugar and may have considerable elevation of blood sugar without showing glycosuria. Routine blood sugar estimation is therefore to be recommended.

Proteinuria can be a useful indicator of urinary infection or renal disease but difficulties arise from false positives due to contamination because of the problems of collecting a true mid-stream specimen in immobile or confused patients. Similarly bacterial contamination is frequent so that quantitative reporting of bacterial growth is necessary if infection is not to be grossly over-diagnosed. Occasionally one may need to resort to suprapubic needle aspiration of the bladder if the clinical importance of a reliable urinary culture results justifies this.

RADIOISOTOPE TESTS

Radioisotope techniques are often of particular value because of their atraumatic nature. Organ scanning techniques may offer considerable advantages in comparison with alternative diagnostic methods because they are less demanding on the ill patient and require less time and cooperation. The brain scan is a minor procedure in comparison with alternative neurosurgical investigations. Computerised tomography is, however, a far more powerful technique which is both more sensitive and better able to distinguish between different cerebral pathologies. The R.I.S.A. scan for non-communicating hydrocephalus is far safer than the alternative air encephalography. Liver scans and lung scans may also be useful, the latter being one of the best methods of confirming the diagnosis of pulmonary embolism, a common diagnostic problem in elderly patients.

Radioisotope thyroid function tests may be used in confirmation of thyroid disease when the screening tests fail to give clear-cut results. I^{125} fibrinogen studies can be valuable in the early detection of thrombo-embolism in geriatric patients (Denham *et al.*, 1972).

ULTRASOUND

Ultrasound offers another non-invasive technique that is particularly suited to investigation of the elderly. It is particularly useful in the investigation of abdominal masses, particularly in visualising the liver, bile ducts and gall bladder.

BONE BIOPSY

This is an important investigation used to confirm the diagnosis of osteomalacia. It is well tolerated by elderly patients when performed under local anaesthesia using a trephine such as the Sacker-Nordin instrument. The specimen is taken from the iliac crest. Until recently the technical difficulties of cutting good undecalcified bone sections which are required for the diagnosis of osteomalacia has tended to limit the full use of bone biopsy. Fortunately, recent work has shown that preliminary silver staining followed by decalcification and normal paraffin sectioning will give equally valid results and is far easier technically so that bone biopsy can now be used far more readily.

NEEDLE BIOPSIES

Needle biopsy techniques are perhaps underused in the investigation of elderly patients and yet are well tolerated procedures. Liver biopsy seems to be particularly neglected and yet can often give valuable information. Similarly needle biopsy of breast lumps is a minor procedure which allows a definite diagnosis to be made.

Further Reading

Caird, F I (1978) Investigation of the elderly patient, Medicine (3rd series), *1*. 15-19.
Hodkinson, H M (1977) Biochemical diagnosis of the elderly, Chapman Hall, London.
Hyams, D E (1980) Nutrition and anaemia, p 100-122, in Metabolic and nutritional disorders in the elderly, Eds. Exton-Smith, A N & Caird, F I, John Wright & Sons Ltd., Bristol.

6

Patterns of Illness in Old Age

Illness in the elderly can be quite different; presentation may be obscure or misleading and the progress and outcome modified. These special features provide much of the interest of geriatric medicine and result in exacting but fascinating diagnostic and management problems.

The challenge is particularly great when illness develops over a considerable time and presents in a non-specific manner. The resulting slow physical, mental or social deterioration is all too easily passed off as due to old age or "senility" and unless full use is made of history taking, examination and appropriate investigation, treatable disease may be missed with tragic consequences.

Unexplained deterioration of any kind must be regarded seriously and as requiring careful diagnosis if the doctor working with the elderly is to care for them adequately. A major educational effort is needed to teach the old, their relatives and all the professional people who deal with the elderly that medical help should be sought for any unexplained deterioration of health or function and that such changes are not to be accepted as a part of normal ageing.

ALTERED PAIN RESPONSE

The key symptom of pain, which is so often the reason why a patient seeks medical help, less commonly results from disease in the old. Even when pain does occur it may be less severe or easily forgotten or the pain is accepted stoically as one of the many burdens of old age. The elderly commonly have considerable difficulty in giving an accurate description of the character and localisation of pain.

Many diseases which are typically associated with pain may be completely painless in old people. Painless myocardial infarction is more common than the classical presentation with severe chest pain and shock. The patient instead presents with the development of heart failure, a minor episode of confusion or a "queer turn" and there may be very little in the clinical picture to point to cardiac pathology as the cause.

Painless vertebral collapse due to osteoporosis is another common situation and the absence of pain or abdominal discomfort in retention of urine may lead to the distended bladder being overlooked.

ALTERED TEMPERATURE RESPONSE

Illness less often results in fever and rigors are very rarely encountered. Urinary infection or pneumonia are often accompanied by a normal temperature, adding to difficulty of diagnosis.

Hypothermia is an important and far from rare accompaniment of severe illness and those dealing with the elderly need to keep the possibility well in mind. Its occurence is not confined to the winter months and it may be met in well-heated hospital wards as well as the spartan unheated bedroom which seems to be an integral part of the way of life of the elderly. The clinical picture is a characteristic one of a drowsy, confused patient with a pale and somewhat myxoedematous general appearance, bradycardia and an abdomen which feels cold to the touch. The superficial resemblance to myxoedema is further strengthened by the presence of "hung-up" tendon reflexes, that is there is considerable delay in the relaxation stage of the reflex. A rectal temperature reading using a low-reading thermometer which is given adequate time to equilibrate is needed to confirm the diagnosis as mouth temperature can be misleading, and a value below 35°C is usually taken as the dividing line (Royal College of Physicians, 1966). Although hypothermia may occur as a result of unusual exposure to cold, justifying the usual term of accidental hypothermia, most cases in the elderly are a consequence of severe illness so that this is something of a misnomer. Prognosis is grave as the dangers of hypothermia, particularly of increased susceptibility to chest infection and of multiple infarctions of viscera, are added to the ill effects of the pre-existing severe illness. Active rewarming is contra-indicated in treatment, the patient should be adequately insulated and allowed to rewarm spontaneously.

MISSING SYMPTOMS

Because of the relative immobility of many elderly patients, symptoms related to exertion may fail to be evoked. Thus angina pectoris and intermittent claudication are encountered far less commonly than would be predicted on the basis of the high prevalence of vascular disease. Similarly patients with severe cardiac or respiratory disease may not complain of exertional dyspnoea.

Sometimes a consequence is that effective treatment of a disabling condition such as Parkinsonism may result in the uncovering of a latent symptom because of the increase in the degree of exertion the patient can undertake.

COMPLICATIONS OF ILLNESS

Mental

The elderly are particularly likely to develop mental manifestations as a complication of their physical illness. The acute confusional state is the most typical response; the mental state is variable, there may be clouding of consciousness and hallucinations as well as confusion and restlessness. The underlying cause may be any severe illness but pneumonia, cardiac failure and urinary infection are particularly commonly to blame (Hodkinson, 1973). Drugs may be responsible, especially barbiturates, tricyclic antidepressants and anti-Parkinsonian drugs. More chronic confusional states may result from such causes as uraemia, carcinomatosis, myxoedema, diabetic pre-coma or pernicious anaemia. Confusional states can occur in intellectually well preserved individuals but pre-existing dementia and also Parkinsonism appear to favour their development. The sudden onset of mental disturbance in a previously normal old person should therefore be recognised as a strong indication that there is an underlying physical basis.

Depression also commonly occurs in the setting of physical illness, particularly in chronic respiratory disease, congestive cardiac failure or after a major stroke. On the other hand uncomplicated depression may present in the guise of physical illness. Hypochondriacal symptoms such as constipation, multiple aches and pains, headaches and giddiness may be prominent and anorexia may result in marked loss of weight.

True or apparent dementia may result from physical disease. Thus deterioration may be due to multiple cerebro-vascular accidents or primary or secondary tumour of the brain. Metabolic mechanisms may be involved as in myxoedema, vitamin B_{12} deficiency, drug intoxications or the dementia that may occur in association with carcinoma without brain secondaries. Sub-dural haematoma and noncommunicating low pressure hydrocephalus are occasional causes which are of special importance because of the possibility of effective treatment.

Physical

The elderly are specially vulnerable to the dangers of confinement to bed. Important among these are the liability to develop bedsores, contractures, foot-drop, constipation, incontinence, stiffening of the joints and loss of balance. Long periods in bed are likely to result in demoralisation of elderly patients and to osteoporosis and muscle wasting as a result of disuse.

Confinement to bed also predisposes to chest infections to which frail elderly patients have an increased susceptibility in any case. Pneumonia remains the "old man's friend" and the outcome of such episodes is little influenced by antibiotic therapy—one of the reasons why life expectation in old age has improved only marginally this century.

Apparently minor intercurrent illness may quite often prove overwhelming in frail and ill old people. A carbuncle may be enough to kill whilst a strain of influenza giving a negligible mortality in other age groups proved highly lethal in geriatric in-patients, those who survived taking many months to fully recover from their set-back, some indeed becoming permanent invalids as a consequence.

Deep vein thrombosis and subsequent pulmonary embolism is another hazard and although bed rest predisposes to it, it may often occur in susceptible patients such as those with stroke or cardiac failure even with a policy of early mobilisation. Many old patients who go downhill for no very obvious reason in fact do so because of pulmonary embolism which is often multiple and may be clinically otherwise silent or merely manifested by a minor "queer turn" or apparent faint.

Dehydration easily develops in ill old people who are unable to fend for themselves and appear to be less likely to experience thirst. As renal impairment is so commonly present, the addition of dehydration readily results in quite marked uraemia. Electrolyte disturbances are also common and the elderly seem particularly prone to the development of hypokalaemia. Osmoregulation seems to be impaired fairly often in severe illness and hypo-osmolality and features of the syndrome of inappropriate secretion of anti-diuretic hormone are not rare.

NON-SPECIFIC PRESENTATIONS

Presentation is frequently vague and ill-defined. Often the clinical picture can be summed up as "failure to thrive". The patient just is not as good as he used to be. He is less able to cope in everyday life, he may lose his edge intellectually and loses interest in eating properly and in outside activities. There may be some weight loss and he may experience tiredness, weakness or malaise with perhaps some minor and ill-defined discomfort or pain. The insidious nature of his illness and the lack of any clear cut symptoms means that the patient may well fail to seek medical help until a late stage is reached or some crisis situation has developed. Even if he does seek medical help at an early stage there is a danger that his doctor may too readily accept his deterioration as merely due to his age.

Unalarming and vague presentations such as this can indicate the development of a great variety of diseases, some serious, many amenable to effective treatment if the correct diagnosis is made, so that the doctor needs to be on his mettle and to make full use of history, examination and investigation.

Malignant disease can present in this way and may be at a late stage with widespread metastasis but even so, in the case of prostatic or breast carcinoma, treatment may have something to offer and useful control may follow the use of stilboestrol. Metabolic disorders also present as "failure to thrive", for example diabetes, uraemia, myxoedema or thyrotoxicosis, and routine screening tests are needed to pick these up reliably. Chronic infections need to be remembered, tuberculosis in the elderly man and sub-acute bacterial endocarditis when there are damaged heart valves. Drugs may be responsible as in the cases of hypokalaemia from long-term diuretic therapy or depression from the prolonged use of reserpine for the control of mild hypertension. Atypical endogenous depression also needs to be considered and direct questioning specifically directed to mood, sleep and appetite may be necessary to reveal this.

Other patients can present with gradual deterioration of mobility or with falls—again a situation which can easily be ascribed to old age itself. Parkinsonism is a cause which is often missed because tremor is absent or unobtrusive; it is a potent cause of both immobility and of falling about. Peripheral neuropathy, which may commonly be due to diabetes, can also be overlooked because of the difficulties of neurological examination in the elderly. There are many other causes of falls; unstable knees, postural hypotension, vertebro-basilar insufficiency, Stokes-Adams attacks, subacute combined degeneration of the cord and "premonitory falls" heralding acute illness such as pneumonia are examples. Painful or deformed feet are another reason for immobility or unsteadiness, arthritic changes, corns and calluses or ingrowing onychogryphoses may all be responsible.

"Rheumatic pains", that is vague generalised musculo-skeletal pain or discomfort, may also indicate serious disease and should not be too readily accepted as due to such osteoarthritis as is present. Causes include bone metastases, especially from lung, breast or prostate, multiple myeloma deposits and osteomalacia. Osteomalacia is an eminently treatable disease which occurs mainly in the housebound, particularly females and those with previous gastric surgery. It results in progressive skeletal pain and proximal muscle weakness which can produce a typical "penguin" gait. Polymyalgia rheumatica, a variant of temporal arteritis, is another disease which responds excellently to treatment (with corticosteroids) and may present with "rheumatic" pains and malaise. It often leads to a very high E.S.R. and can be confirmed by temporal artery biopsy.

MASKING BY KNOWN DISEASES

One unfortunate consequence of multiple disease is that the symptoms and signs of a new disease may be wrongly attributed to the old diseases already diagnosed. Patients with extensive osteoarthritis or rheumatoid arthritis who have multiple falls may sustain a fracture of the femoral neck which is over-looked because the pain and immobility can be readily explained as due to exacerbation of the arthritis. Osteomalacia too can readily be missed in arthritic patients. An increase in the cardiac failure of a patient with long diagnosed valvular heart disease may be due to a new development such as thyrotoxicosis or subacute bacterial endocarditis. Patients themselves may ascribe their present symptoms to their old diseases so the physician must avoid being misled and should always consider the possibility of new additional diagnoses.

Further Reading

Hodkinson, H M (1980) Common symptoms of disease in the elderly, 2nd edition, Blackwell Scientific Publications, Oxford.
Simpson, R G (1974) Disease patterns in the elderly, British Journal of Hospital Medicine, 12, 660-667.

7

Care of the Elderly

PRESENT FACTS ABOUT THE ELDERLY

The elderly over 65 now form more than 13% of the population of Great Britain. Approximately one third of the total are over 75. Females, who comprise 51% of the whole population, show an increasing numerical preponderance at higher ages, outnumbering men by 58% over 65, by two to one over 75 and by three to one over 85. The female of 65 has an average life expectation of 16 years compared to 12 years for the male, at 75 she has 9½ years compared to 7 and at 85 has 5 years compared to 4.

Something like 95 per cent of the elderly live at home whilst only about 5 per cent are cared for in institutions. An approximate breakdown is that of every nine people over 65 in the community, three live with their spouse, two live alone, two live with an unmarried child, one with a married child and one with a more distant relative, friend or companion. Of those in institutional care, roughly half are in homes, mainly those run by local authorities, and half in hospitals (about two-fifths in geriatric departments). These figures are for those over 65 but it is the most elderly who make the heaviest use of institutional resources. Those over 75 provide the bulk of the work of geriatric departments, usually forming about three-quarters of the total. The majority of medical admissions for patients over 75 are to geriatric beds whilst only a minority of the 65-74 age-group are dealt with. Many females in the highest age-groups outlive husbands, siblings and contemporaries and become socially isolated and vulnerable. Even minor illness can result in a major emergency because it may be impracticable to provide sufficient help to allow the period of illness to be coped with at home and hospital admission is therefore required.

CARE OF THE ELDERLY IN THE COMMUNITY

The Family. As some two-thirds of the elderly live with relatives, support from the family is a factor of great importance in practical terms. The extent of the help given by families to their old relatives is often remarkable. Patients with major mental and physical disability who are receiving long-term care in geriatric and psychiatric departments are outnumbered by many old people who are equally severely incapacitated and yet are cared for in their own homes with devotion and often considerable self sacrifice by their families.

31

Although families are smaller in size than they were in the past, fewer children available to help may not be a real disadvantage as it is possibly balanced by closer bonds between parent and child. All too often one finds that in a very large family each child feels that one of the many others should take on the responsibility of caring for the aged parent, and not themselves. Typically it is the unmarried child, often a younger daughter who has never left home, who is obliged to assume the main burden of responsibility for the parent. This will perhaps be less so in the future in the light of present higher marriage rates and this is perhaps fortunate as, while the parent living with a single child is a common situation, it is often not a satisfactory one. There may be strong bonds of affection, but it is common for the daughter to feel resentment and aggression at the same time and for the interplay of these contrary emotions to give rise to guilt. The parent may sense these tensions and react by being excessively demanding or critical. All too often, parent and child come to invest the major part of their emotional capital in this one relationship and excessive and thwarting interdependence develops. Brocklehurst and Shergold (1968) indeed found that discharge of an elderly patient from hospital was most often resented by the unmarried child to whom they returned as compared to married children or to their spouse (resentment being rare in the latter case).

Living with married children involves rather different problems such as conflict with the in-law or arguments over the upbringing of the grand-children but the parent and married child usually avoid the perils of the special emotional intensity and interdependence which typify the relationship with the unmarried child. The better success usually seen where parent lives with married child may also be because there is more of an element of choice for both parties so that resentment, guilt and mere duty play a smaller part to the benefit of all concerned.

Outsiders can often be quick in condemnation of the exceptional case where children refuse to help a parent in need. Unreasonable refusal is in fact most uncommon (Isaacs, 1971) and many refusals are based on compelling reason if one takes the trouble to investigate the circumstances. The elderly parent who is rejected has all too often rejected the child in the past. The family cupboard may be found to contain unpleasant skeletons such as alcoholism, violence, abandonment, desertion, sexual aberrations or infidelities, illegitimacy or crime. When one knows the details, rejection is not surprising. What may be surprising is the capacity of some children to rise above such past events and give help to an aged parent which is thoroughly undeserved.

The Elderly Living Alone. Those living alone may have children but may, even if somewhat incapacitated, prefer to maintain their own independent way of life rather than accept an offer to go to live with them. They may feel, perhaps quite correctly, that their relationship with their children would not stand up satisfactorily to the pressures of living in the same household. Their relatives may none the less provide a great deal of help by frequent visiting but this depends on reasonable proximity. Unfortunately modern social mobility often scatters families widely and may mean that children are too far away to help effectively.

With no relatives at hand, friends and neighbours can be a powerful source of help and quite severely disabled old people may maintain some sort of independence in their own home with the assistance they give. Some old people, although showing admirable determination to continue to live in their own home, may fail to realise or accept that they are laying a very heavy burden on those who are responsible for helping them. In such situations where the lack of insight of the old person becomes apparent, it may be tempting to over-persuade or coerce them to give up their home and go to live with a relative or enter an old people's home. This can lead to great unhappiness and prolonged resentment if the old person does not accept the decision as truly being his own and feels that he was forced to make it. The elderly need to feel that they can decide their own future for themselves and should be allowed to take risks or live in a squalid and apparently unsatisfactory way if others are not seriously affected by their decision. The temptation to project ones own standards and expectations onto the elderly must be resisted and they must not be pushed into "tidy" solutions against their wishes so as to salve the consciences or ease the anxieties of others.

Housing. The ability of the elderly to live successfully in their own home is very much affected by their housing. The old may often cope well despite the fact that they live in apparently grossly inadequate housing which may be too large for their present needs. It may be old, damp and in poor decorative and structural repair and have too many stairs and poorly lit passages. Heating, lighting, cooking and sanitary facilities may seem appallingly old-fashioned and inconvenient. They cope well because the house is familiar and because it is in a long settled community where they know their neighbours and have many local friends and acquaintances so that they have a rich network of social interaction and of people on whom they can call for support and help. Rehousing in some apparently ideal specially designed and physically far superior accommodation can be an unmitigated disaster because of unfamiliarity and the breaking of all their old social ties by a move of perhaps only a few hundred yards. Modern tower blocks of flats are particularly likely to isolate and demoralise the elderly who are rehoused within them.

The common practice of moving house to a new town on retirement may also sow the seeds of later disaster. Relatives and friends are left behind and congregation of the elderly in retirement areas, such as the south coast resorts, results in enormous strains on local services for the elderly because of the severe distortion of the population structure with a third or more over retirement age.

Sheltered housing, usually in the form of warden flatlets, has much to commend it and may offer great advantages to the old person who is having difficulty in coping in his old accommodation but is keen to preserve as much independence as possible and neither needs nor wishes to accept the greater degree of care provided in an old people's home. In many ways warden flatlets are a modern equivalent of the almshouses of the past. They should be sited near to the former homes of the residents and with easy access by public transport. They consist of a group of perhaps twenty or so flatlets which are especially designed for the needs of one or two old people. There is a resident warden who can check that each resident is all right each day and will call assistance when it is needed. The warden is not expected to provide domestic or nursing assistance. There is commonly some communal accommodation and activity so that a sense of belonging to a community can be developed. Warden flatlets have proved to be of real value and increasing numbers are being built by local authorities.

Social services for the elderly

Social services for the elderly are mainly provided by the local authority but a variety of voluntary organisations provide additional services in many areas.

Home Helps. This is a most important local authority service which deals principally with the old. Home Helps work in the old person's own home for a set number of hours per week and there is a charge according to means. The Home Help undertakes usual household tasks such as cleaning, dusting, bed-making, shopping and errands, cooking and washing. She is not intended to give nursing attention.

Many disabled elderly people should ideally have help each day but in many areas this is not often possible because of the many calls on the service. Home Helps are typically mature women with great sympathy and interest in their elderly clients and can very easily become a key figure in the old person's life. Close ties may develop and it is not uncommon to find that the Home Help does far more than she is strictly required to do and may make extra visits to do little extra jobs or to see that all is well. During illness they may unofficially take on nursing duties and many an old person, who would otherwise need to be admitted to hospital, is kept at home thanks to their willingness.

A development arising out of the success of the Home Help Service is the introduction of the "friendly neighbour" scheme whereby a willing local person can receive some small renumeration in return for regular visiting to help an incapacitated old person.

Meals on Wheels. This is another key service which was pioneered by voluntary bodies but has now been adopted by local authorities. Many old people lack the motivation or the ability to cook adequate meals for themselves. If they are frail or housebound they are unable to avail themselves of the meals that may be provided at old people's clubs or to make use of restaurants or cafes. Meals on wheels fill an important gap, delivering a hot cooked lunch to the old person's own table at low cost. Disadvantages are that it may not be possible to provide a meal each day because of the heavy demands on the service and that most services are not able to provide meals suitable for those on therapeutic diets such as diabetics.

Social Activities. Loneliness is a common problem, particularly for the housebound. Friendly visiting on a regular basis is organised by many voluntary societies and they run many clubs which are suitable for the more active who are able to get about out of doors.

Day centres are provided by local authorities but their success depends on the provision of special transport so that the housebound and frail are able to attend. Day centres can provide a full day of activity including a mid-day meal and attendance may also be useful to relieve a relative who is otherwise completely tied.

Laundry Service. Local authorities may provide an incontinent laundry service to assist those who are looking after an incontinent patient in the home. In addition disposable incontinence pads can now be provided.

Holidays. Relatives may care for incapacitated old people for long periods without complaint and with no outside help but then find that they can never take a holiday because of the commitment. They can be helped in a number of ways. It may be possible to arrange for the old person to have a holiday; many voluntary bodies make such arrangements or, if a general practitioner considers it could benefit health, a recuperative holiday through the local authority can be obtained. However many old people may be too frail or ill for such arrangements. Most local authorities provide short term "holiday admissions" to their old peoples homes for frail ambulant old people. Where the old person is too incapacitated or ill for this there is usually an equivalent service offered by the local geriatric service whereby the patient is booked for a two week admission to cover the holiday period.

Professional Services for the Elderly in the Community

Home Nursing. The District Nurses, working under the direction of the general practitioner, devote much of their time to the care of the elderly at home. They usually make brief visits and are particularly involved in technical procedures such as injections, dressings to ulcers and enemas. Bathing helpless old patients is another common requirement. The District Nurse may also advise relatives on how to nurse the old patient and can help to arrange for nursing equipment such as urinals, commodes, waterproof sheets or hoists to be temporarily borrowed.

The Health Visitor. Health Visitors are trained nurses who have undergone further training in the social aspects of illness and preventive health. Increasingly they are involving themselves in the community care of the elderly but in an advisory, supportive and follow-up role rather than a nursing capacity. They are often active in the ascertainment of need which is so important in effective care of the elderly and in furtherance of this they are developing links with general practice and with hospital geriatric departments through a variety of attachment arrangements.

Social Workers. Social workers are employed by the local authority and may work either in the community or in hospital. A key role is to ascertain the wishes of the old person with respect to his future. Where these are unrealistic much counselling and discussion may be needed to try to modify the old person's views but these cannot be over-ruled for the well motivated individual may well succeed against apparently overwhelming odds. In the community the social worker acts as an indispensable link between the client and the confusing array of different services which are available to help them. They have special responsibility for groups of disabled old people such as the blind, deaf and mentally or physically handicapped.

The General Practitioner. The General Practitioner holds a key position in the provision of care for the elderly in the community. Practically all old people are registered with a general practitioner and he is the only doctor directly available to them for help and advice. The G.P. spends a good deal of his total time with his elderly patients because of their greater vulnerability and this is recognised by the payment of a higher capitation fee for elderly patients on his list. With his experience and local knowledge, the G.P. has much to give to his elderly patients; he can mobilise help in many ways and many statutory services are provided on his authority.

Other Professions. Domiciliary chiropody for the housebound is a valued service in view of the prevalence of foot pathology such as corns, calluses and nail defects but lack of available personnel often detracts from the adequacy of the service.

Many local authorities now employ occupational therapists who can assess problems in the home and give appropriate advice or arrange for the provision of various aids or adaptations to the house such as handrails, ramps or more practicable sanitary arrangements.

Pilot schemes for the provision of domiciliary physiotherapy have been tried in some areas but have not yet become firmly established.

Residential Care of the Elderly

Welfare Homes (old people's homes) are provided by the local authority and residents in them pay according to their means. Welfare homes are intended for old people who are unable to live independently in their own home even with the help of social services and need more assistance than is available in sheltered housing. Residents need to be ambulant at least with aids, should not need more than minor help with dressing, should be continent at least during the day and their mental state should be good enough for them to be suitable for care in the home and to fit into its communal life. Their medical care remains the responsibility of their general practitioner.

The oldest welfare homes, converted from former poor-law accommodation, have now thankfully been largely replaced but there remain post-war homes which were conversions of large houses which often provide less than ideal resources, particularly as a lift may be lacking so that many residents have to climb stairs. The majority of homes are now more recent buildings specifically designed as homes and these have lifts and other desirable resources to allow them to cope with the many frail residents who need care. These modern homes typically have places for about fifty residents and their superintendent and deputy superintendent often have nursing training or experience.

There is usually a considerable waiting list for welfare home and assessment of suitability and priority for admission of applicants is one of the tasks of the local authority social workers. In addition to the local authority homes, there are independent homes run either by voluntary organisations or for profit (voluntary homes and rest homes). These may be smaller and more homely and also offer the elderly some degree of choice if they have sufficient means. Voluntary homes often cater for some specific group, occupational, professional or religious, and this bond of common interest may help to foster a better sense of community and belonging than is possible in other homes where backgrounds and interests vary more widely. The merits, differences and problems of the various types of homes for the elderly have been penetratingly examined in "The Last Refuge" (Townsend, 1962) a book which is essential reading for anyone with a serious interest in the elderly.

HOSPITAL CARE OF THE ELDERLY

The elderly are admitted to many different hospital departments such as surgical departments, especially orthopaedics, and the full range of medical specialties. It is only beyond the age of 75 that the majority of medical admissions are to departments of geriatric medicine.

The general features of patients selected for admission to geriatric departments were outlined in Chapter 1 but in summary they are the very elderly, those with multiple problems and those where the need for rehabilitation or of long-term care is anticipated.

The Geriatric Department. Geriatric departments serve a defined catchment area and are usually comparatively large in size, most commonly with around two-hundred beds. Present policy in Britain is that at least half of the beds should be within the local District General Hospital but this has yet to be generally achieved and some departments may still be completely without such beds and correspondingly be at risk of isolation from the rest of hospital medical activity.

Most departments adopt some sort of scheme of progressive patient care. Typically admission and assessment wards are within the District General Hospital and all patients are admitted through them. Here they can receive full medical, psychiatric and social assessment and make use of the full investigational and therapeutic resources that are available. Patients, other than those for whom only a short stay is needed, may then be transferred on to rehabilitation and intermediate care wards which may also be within the District General Hospital but sometimes in a nearby hospital. Here treatment can be continued with particular emphasis on active rehabilitation and eventual return home. Not all patients are capable of improving sufficiently for their discharge home, however, and when this is the case patients are transferred to long-stay wards which are commonly in small local hospitals, often former fever or tuberculosis hospitals. Long-stay wards need to be regarded as the patient's home for the rest of his life and so staff must make special efforts to ensure that there is a happy and homely atmosphere and that visiting is made as easy as is possible. At the same time the highest standards of nursing care need to be maintained and doctors must continue to take a proper interest in their irremediable patients. Provided that these points are remembered and that the physical resources of the wards are brought up to modern standards, these small long-stay hospital units can function very satisfactorily and it is not then necessary, as has sometimes been recommended, that all geriatric beds should be provided on the main hospital site. There is a danger, however, that if too many of a department's beds are long-stay beds in such units, which are isolated and without full hospital facilities, the excess of long-stay beds will tend to create an excess of long-stay patients to fill them.

Admission to the Geriatric Department. Geriatric departments admit elderly patients who need *hospital* as opposed to residential care such as can be provided in a welfare home. Most departments do not deal with physically fit, mentally disturbed patients whose hospital care is the responsibility of the psychogeriatric service, or of the psychiatric service where a specialised service for the elderly has not been instituted. However, geriatric departments do deal with many old people with psychiatric disturbance when this is in the setting of physical illness or disability.

Admission arrangements vary considerably from one department to another, a major distinction being whether or not there is a waiting list. Unfortunately many departments do have a sizable waiting list for admission and so feel the need to vet applications for admission very carefully to determine priority or to avoid admission completely. Most such departments employ routine domiciliary assessment visiting to this end, the visits being made by a doctor from the department, sometimes accompanied by a social worker. Routine visiting can take up an enormous amount of staff time and energies, tends to delay the admission of the old person in urgent need of admission and may be seen by general practitioners as indicating a lack of trust in their capacity for assessing their own patients. The visits do confer the benefits of intimate knowledge of the patient's home situation and may help to establish a close rapport with him.

Other departments find that, by maintaining a higher turnover of patients through the beds of the unit, a waiting list can be avoided (Hodkinson and Jefferys, 1972) and that most patients can be admitted without any special assessment by the department staff but using the general practitioner's appraisal of the situation. The patient is usually admitted without delay on the same day when the need for admission is clear-cut. If the general practitioner has any doubts about the usefulness of admission he can make use of domiciliary consultation or out-patient attendance to obtain specialist geriatric advice.

All departments take a proportion of their admissions by transfer from other departments (commonly some 15 per cent or so), patients being accepted when they are in need of the special expertise or resources of the department, such as rehabilitation or the provision of long-stay care.

Outcome for Patients who are Admitted. The majority of patients admitted to a geriatric department are subsequently discharged to their own homes but a small proportion may be placed in old people's homes or private accommodation. The chances of discharge are much the same for the two sexes as Fig. 3 illustrates. It can also be seen that the majority of discharges occur after a fairly short time in hospital, most within the first two months, so that prolonged stay in hospital is a feature of only a small proportion of elderly admissions.

A waiting list can have adverse effects on the patient's discharge potential as deterioration may occur during the wait and additional complications such as pressure sores develop. Morale may suffer and relatives and general practitioner may prove less cooperative in arranging the discharge if they had a long wait for admission and fear its repetition should readmission later prove necessary.

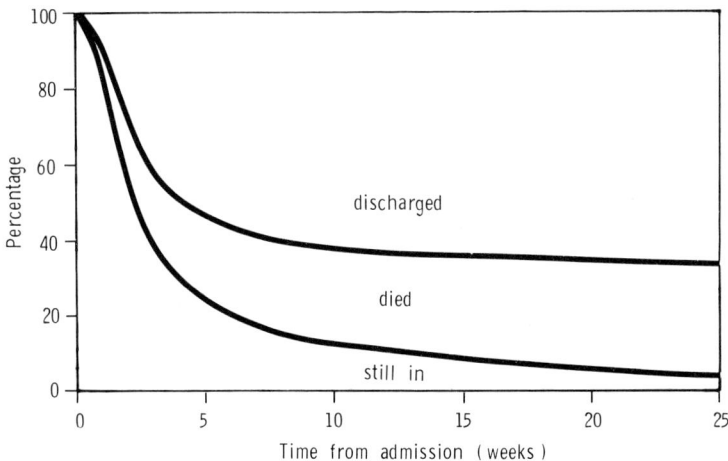

Fig. 3 (a). Outcome of consecutive admissions of men to a department of geriatric medicine (from Hodkinson and Hodkinson, 1980).

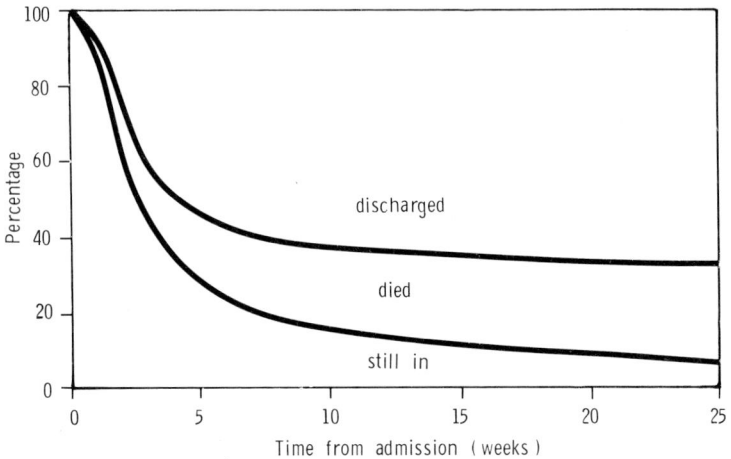

Fig. 3 (b). Outcome of consecutive admissions of women to a department of geriatric medicine (from Hodkinson and Hodkinson, 1980).

Many geriatric patients are very ill when admitted and some are specifically taken in for terminal care. Hospital mortality is thus understandably high and is particularly concentrated in the early weeks after admission (Fig. 3). There is a considerable sex difference, males having a substantially higher death rate.

Discharge from Hospital. The discharge of the elderly patient from hospital calls for careful planning and teamwork. The holding of multidisciplinary case conferences in association with ward rounds has now become a standard practice in departments of geriatric medicine. Here, doctors, nurses, therapists and social workers involved in the patient's care can exchange information and opinions and arrive at well formulated decisions. Home visits by the patient and his therapists may give important additional information and perhaps allow home modifications to be initiated in good time or clarify treatment aims. The role of the social worker is of particular importance, ensuring that the patient's wishes are taken into proper account. She communicates with relatives and friends to secure their support and understanding and she plans ahead so that social arrangements, which may well be complicated, can be brought to fruition in good time and not be responsible for frustrating delay of discharge. She is directly involved in the arrangements for provision of social services such as home help and meals on wheels and also makes all the arrangements for admission to a welfare home if this is necessary.

After-care. Many geriatric departments have a specific geriatric health visitor who attends case conferences and can ensure that, where appropriate, there is close follow-up during the critical early days or weeks following discharge, checking that the arrangements that have been made are functioning effectively, monitoring the patient's progress and enlisting further help should it be needed. She can also guide the patient and relatives so that rehabilitation gains are maintained, rather than a pattern of unnecessary dependence becoming re-established because of over-protective attitudes. The patient's general practitioner is vitally concerned in the successful discharge from hospital. He must be kept fully informed and must have all the relevant information about his newly discharged patient without delay if he is to give effective support. Without such support and supervision, which are particularly necessary in the early days and weeks after discharge, patients can very easily relapse and all the benefits of the hospital admission be lost.

The Geriatric Day Hospital. The geriatric day hospital may be used to support the patient following his discharge. However there are inherent disadvantages as continued hospital attendance can result in further institutionalisation and there is some risk of displacing the general practitioner from his central role in caring for the patient at home. Day hospital care has a clearly useful role when follow-up at home has shown some loss of independence since discharge. A "refresher course" of rehabilitation may quickly retrieve the situation and is a far more efficient use of resources than the open-ended continuation of "maintenance therapy" after discharge.

In-patient or Day Hospital Care. The need for in-patient care for severely ill elderly patients may often be unarguable but there are less pressing situations where the balance of advantage between in-patient and day hospital care need careful consideration.

Hospital admission has quite definite risks, Rosin and Boyd (1966) showing that a good half of old people may develop complications which are not obviously related to the cause for admission but may be due to admission itself. Confusion, pressure sores and incontinence are well recognised hazards. Hospital admission may also result in institutionalisation and demoralisation of the elderly, despite one's best efforts to avoid these effects. Patients may come to fear their discharge home increasingly so that successful return to independent life becomes a fight against time. Well judged compromise may be necessary if the slowing rate of physical improvement achieved by continued hospital stay is not to be more than offset by progressively increasing demoralisation.

Clearly hospital admission may have much to offer also. Its concentration of medical, investigational, rehabilitation and nursing resources is often indispensable and leaves no alternative for the management of the elderly patient. Day hospital may be a practical alternative to admission for some patients, particularly when the need is principally for rehabilitation but the degree of incapacity is not too great. When admission is not urgent there is also the opportunity to prepare the patient by thorough explanation of the aims and likely course of hospital stay and thus to minimise the demoralising effects.

Psychogeriatric Care. Separate psychogeriatric services are being set up in many areas to deal principally with depressive illness and with disturbed but physically healthy patients with dementia. These are at present mainly based on the large mental hospitals but this does not prevent the creation of effective and active departments. In the future it is likely that services may be based on smaller hospitals in the community which will have close links with the geriatric and psychiatric services within the District General Hospital. Many of the less disturbed patients who in the past were admitted to mental hospitals will increasingly be cared for in suitable welfare homes provided by local authorities.

Day care can play a major role in the provision of psychogeriatric care and both day hospitals and local authority day centres are of proven worth.

Further Reading

Brearly, C P (1975) Social work, ageing and society, Routledge & Kegan Paul, London.

Brocklehurst, J C & Tucker, J S (1980) Progress in geriatric day care, King Edward's Hospital Fund for London, London.

Evans, J. G. (1978) Demography and resources, Medicine (3rd series), *1*, 12-14.

Hunt, A (1978) The elderly at home, H.M.S.O., London.

Jefferys, M (1978) The elderly in society, p 763-782, in Textbook of geriatric medicine and gerontology, Ed. Brocklehurst, J C, Churchill Livingstone, Edinburgh.

Townsend, P (1962) The last refuge, Routledge & Kegan Paul, London.

8

Rehabilitation of the Elderly

Rehabilitation, the achievement of the optimum level of independence for the individual, is particularly important in geriatric work. This is because specific disabilities calling for rehabilitation, such as hemiplegia, parkinsonism, arthritis, fracture or amputation, are particularly common in the aged but also because any illness necessitating a period of inactivity may lead to increased dependency and loss of the abilities for self-care and mobility in a frail old person.

Bed rest has dangers in any age group as so clearly described by Asher (1947). It is especially likely to have ill effects in the elderly. Bed rest must be minimised because of its adverse effects on confidence, balance, mobility and joint stiffness but where it cannot be avoided these penalties mean that a period of rehabilitation must follow to undo the damage.

Traditional patterns of hospital care involved over-reliance on bed rest and were poorly suited to the needs of the elderly in other respects. The institutionalisation of elderly patients was a common consequence of attitudes which cast the patient too much in the role of the passive recipient of care and demanded of him only grateful acceptance of that care. His status as patient rather than person was reinforced by the substitution of slippers and dressing gown for everyday clothing and polite subservience by uniforms, ranks and hierarchies. These influences are all too likely to result in a patient who is over anxious to conform and to say to the doctor "you know best, I leave it all to you".

The requirements for effective rehabilitation are diametrically opposite for it is a psychological more than a physical process and the patient's individuality and drive needs to be stimulated not suppressed. The successful outcome of rehabilitation owes more to mental factors than to the degree or nature of the physical disability. Good motivation may lead to recovery even in the face of daunting physical problems whilst poor motivation, depression, anxiety, confusion or dementia may be insuperable barriers to recovery even when the physical disability is relatively minor.

THE THERAPEUTIC ENVIRONMENT

The key to successful rehabilitation is thus the creation of a therapeutic environment which can support and encourage the patient's will to get better and which surrounds him with an atmosphere of hope and positive expectations. Much is said and written about the "rehabilitation team" in this effort but, while physiotherapists, occupational therapists, speech therapists, nurses and social workers who form this team are of great importance, the equal importance of a much wider "supporters club" in producing the required environment must be stressed. That is to say that the patient is significantly influenced by everyone with whom he comes in contact during his hospital stay. His fellow patients, relatives and visitors, orderlies and domestics, porters, chaplains, voluntary workers and staff of other hospital departments may all play a part in determining the quality of the therapeutic environment as well as the doctors and rehabilitation team.

It is crucial that we get this therapeutic environment right. If we do, the geriatric department then offers considerable advantages to the elderly patient in comparison to the other departments which are less well geared to his rehabilitation needs. Medical staff carry a major responsibility and their leadership and enthusiasm are essential contributions. Nurses too may make or mar the quality of the atmosphere, their intimate contact with patients around the clock putting them in a particularly effective position of influence. More senior nurses who were trained in the traditional approach may find the need to make quite considerable readjustments in caring for the elderly. A policy of helping the patient to help himself must replace more custodial attitudes. Habits of over-protection also need to be discarded so that, for example, the necessary risks of allowing patients to walk alone at the appropriate stage of their rehabilitation are accepted rather than inhibiting their progress by remarks such as "don't do that on your own, you might fall". Nurses need to keep themselves well in touch with the progress of their patients' rehabilitation if they are not to fall prey to the wily ones who enjoy the dependent role and seek to prolong it. The common pitfalls are dressing the old patient who dressed herself in occupational therapy and hauling the patient from a chair and walking him with maximum help when he can get up and walk without help when supervised by the physiotherapist.

Effective communication between staff is an essential, not just to avoid this sort of try-on, but so as to create for the patient the reassurance of a unified and consistent therapeutic attitude from all the staff with whom he comes into contact. Staff must also communicate with the patients and relatives and deliberately instil these attitudes and expectations. A particularly important opportunity is at the time of the patient's admission when doctors and the ward sister in particular have to deal with the patient's and relatives' needs for information and reassurance. Beyond this all staff need to take every available opportunity to reinforce the rehabilitation message. Only if these efforts are made will the therapeutic environment be properly established and the essential qualities of enthusiasm and purposive optimism be disseminated and reinforced throughout the whole of the group of people concerned in it.

Deeds are important as well as words and seeing other patients improve and go home is a powerful influence in modifying the generally pessimistic expectations of the elderly and their relatives. In this the more active departments have an advantage. Progressive patient-care systems also help as the segregation of long-stay patients maintains a greater momentum and better rehabilitation atmosphere in the active wards. It is similarly important for the ward to appear to be a dynamic and busy place. A geriatric day room where a drowsy and bored group of patients sit in chairs neatly arranged around the walls and gaze blankly into space is destructive to the morale of patients and staff alike. Efforts should be made to ensure that the ward is instead an active and stimulating place. Social activity needs to be supported by easy visiting arrangements, making use of voluntary workers to encourage social interaction, using games, craft activities, art classes and grouping patients in such a way as to encourage conversation. It can also be an advantage if most of the rehabilitation treatments are on the ward and not away in the particular departments so that the ward benefits from the general increase in activity. Group work may also be of help and may confer social as well as strictly therapeutic benefits.

ENCOURAGEMENT OF THE INDIVIDUAL PATIENT

The individual patient needs personal attention and encouragement as well as the support of a sound therapeutic environment. He needs to establish relationships with his nurses, therapists and doctors to sustain and encourage him and they on their part need to recognise the importance of this: indeed the effectiveness of members of the rehabilitation team relies much more on their use of their own personality than on techniques. He needs them to talk to him, to recognise his individuality and to treat him as a thinking person with a past and a future, not like a mindless pet. The patient needs sympathy without it being overdone and may equally need the challenge of the more ambitious expectations of staff. He needs recognition and praise of success but also help in coming to terms with his failures. He needs to feel valued and may appreciate the reassurance of physical contact such as the arm around the shoulder.

ASSESSMENT OF AIMS

The individual's own wishes regarding his future have a special importance and it can be very hazardous to attempt to overrule strongly held views even when these appear unrealistic. The danger of overpersuasion is that fierce determination and high motivation may be replaced by resentment or apathy. It may be better to accept the patient's own goal and help him to achieve it even though this may mean perhaps his return to a far from ideal home situation or the opposition of neighbours or relatives who are concerned about the risks or low standards involved. On the other hand, the patient's own future plans may be so unrealistic that the task of persuading him to accept alternatives, such as admission to a welfare home as opposed to return to his own home, must be undertaken. This may call for great tact but also firmness as well as sympathy in helping him adjust to the inevitable without catastrophic deterioration in morale. The special skills of the social worker may be invaluable in such situations.

ASSESSMENT OF THE PATIENT

A realistic rehabilitation programme for the individual patient must be based on a thorough assessment of mental, functional, physical and social factors.

The use of a simple questionnaire test of orientation and memory (Hodkinson, 1972) to assess intellectual ability has already been considered. A poor test score, however, need not necessarily mean that rehabilitation will be unsuccessful. Personality and motivation are also very important and, where they are good, even quite severely confused patients may make good progress. It is very important to recognise depression which is a serious obstacle to rehabilitation if left untreated.

The aim of functional assessment is to determine the patient's capabilities for mobility and self care. We also need to know what levels of ability will be required for the patient to resume an independent life. Common basic needs in this respect, the so called "activities of daily living" (A.D.L.) include the ability to walk, get in and out of chair or bed, dress, feed oneself, attend to personal toilet needs and in addition a varying number of other activities such as cooking, housework and climbing stairs. The patient's mental state and continence are other key factors in determining ability to cope back in the community.

Physical assessment will pay particular regard to central nervous system and locomotor abnormalities affecting mobility of A.D.L. skills but also needs to consider other factors. Obesity is a common extra disability, often coupled with osteoarthritis, and weight reduction may be an essential part of the overall rehabilitation scheme. Poor exercise tolerance due to respiratory or cardiac disease may also be an important limiting factor and dyspnoea and a rise in pulse rate to over 130/min. during rehabilitation procedures are crude guides to exercise limits.

Social assessment is an essential basis of a realistic rehabilitation programme with clearly defined aims. Many individuals may be involved in the collection of the relevant facts and it is vital that all the items of information are brought together. This is another example of the importance of communication between members of the rehabilitation staff which can be facilitated by such organisational measures as specific rehabilitation ward rounds or case conferences at which staff can come together to exchange information about patients and their progress.

RESOURCES OF THE REHABILITATION WARD

Rehabilitation of the elderly does not make much use of special equipment other than simple walking aids such as walking frames, tripods and sticks. Crutches are little used as old people have great difficulty balancing with them and usually do far better using a walking frame as an alternative. Adequate space for walking practice is essential and there needs to be sufficient day-room space to allow social and diversional activities to flourish. Floor coverings in the ward need to be non-slip; their appearance is also relevant for old people may be fearful of falling if the floor looks shiny and slippery even though it may be non-slip. Handrails should be provided generously in rooms and corridors and grab rails fitted in toilets and bathrooms to assist getting up. Doors should be light enough to be managed safely by frail old patients and wide enough to admit wheelchairs or hoists. The ward will also need a generous number of geriatric chairs, that is chairs with arms and a range of designs and seat heights suitable for the varying needs of individual patients. Beds should ideally all be of adjustable height so that patients can get in and out unaided with the bed low whilst the bed can be raised for nursing procedures and bed-making. As patients wear their own clothes and shoes during rehabilitation, special geriatric lockers with wardrobe space are of great value. Wheelchairs are also needed but their over-use should be guarded against; nursing convenience should not deprive patients of valuable opportunities for walking practice.

ROLE OF THE MEMBERS OF THE REHABILITATION TEAM

The Physiotherapist

The prospects of discharge of a patient are principally determined by the achievement of independent mobility. This is the physiotherapist's main concern and underlines her importance in the team. Retraining of mobility may need to proceed through stages involving the regaining of sitting and then standing balance before actual ambulation can be attempted. The patient needs to be instructed how to get in and out of his chair safely and how to use walking aids correctly. Patients with specific disorders such as hemiplegia may require highly specialised rehabilitation techniques and need a very heavy investment of the physiotherapist's time. In other patients walking rehabilitation may be very much more straightforward, for example in patients who have become immobile after a period of bed rest whilst acutely ill. Here the physiotherapist can instruct other staff, particularly nursing staff, in the appropriate retraining techniques so that they too can play an active part in the patient's rehabilitation.

Where the patient's disabilities preclude the regaining of the ability to walk, the physiotherapist will train the patient to use a wheelchair. This will involve close cooperation with the occupational therapist, indeed throughout rehabilitation work there is need for sensible overlapping and coordination of activities and no place for rigid attitudes or "demarcation disputes" over who does what.

Another important function of the physiotherapist is in the prevention of contractures. Prevention mainly depends on putting the joints at risk through a full range of movement regularly, a task which the patient may be able to do for himself once he has been suitably instructed or in which nursing staff can be usefully involved. Plastic or plaster of Paris splinting, usually in the form of night splints may sometimes be necessary.

Retraining in climbing stairs is another important task. Oddly, the difficulty of stair climbing for old people is often overestimated. Those with poor balance who walk poorly on the level may perform surprisingly well on stairs where they have the support of handrails.

Throughout their work with elderly patients, physiotherapists are concerned with improvement of function, not with mere muscle power or range of movement. The personality of the individual therapist is the most important therapeutic weapon.

The Occupational Therapist

The principal function of the occupational therapist is in the assessment of the activities of daily living and the retraining of the patient to regain the required competence in them. The areas most often calling for attention are dressing, feeding, getting in and out of bed, bathing, cooking and personal toilet. For many old patients simple checking, practice and encouragement may be all that are needed within the A.D.L. unit of the occupational therapy department. Others may need more specific assistance, either having to learn new ways, as with the hemiplegic who must learn to do many tasks one handed, or requiring the assistance of alterations or gadgets. Difficulty with buttons may therefore call for their replacement by zips or by velcro fastenings whilst difficulty putting on stockings may be overcome by a stocking device. The occupational therapist can often work most usefully in close collaboration with others. Her expertise can be useful in working with the nursing staff when a patient has feeding or dressing problems. The physiotherapist may link up with the occupational therapist when she finds the need for repetitive exercises to improve strength or mobility; some occupational therapy activity such as work on a loom or printing press may provide a far more interesting way of carrying out the required exercise. Most patients abandon exercises such as quadriceps drill the moment the physiotherapist's back is turned but will happily exercise their legs by pedalling when using a machine to make something.

The diversional aspect of occupational therapy has suffered from being overstressed in the past. None the less, diversional activities both in the department and on the ward can play a very real part in stimulating patients and improving their morale.

The Speech Therapist

The speech therapist will be specifically involved in the rehabilitation of the patient who has communication problems. Most commonly she will need to treat patients with neurological disorders resulting in dysphasia, dysarthria or dyspraxia and will concern herself with reading and writing abilities as well as speaking. Apart from individual treatment, she can play an important wider role in education of other staff and relatives in the best ways to assist patients to achieve their full communication potential when disabled by disorders of voice, speech, language or hearing. She can also advise on the psychological handling of patients who are so disabled, as adverse psychological reactions are a common accompaniment of communication difficulties.

The Nurse

The geriatric nurse must be fully involved in her patient's rehabilitation and needs to know what members of the rehabilitation team can do and are doing if she is to collaborate effectively. Particularly relevant areas are dressing and feeding where liaison with the occupational therapist can be most fruitful. In the case of feeding difficulties, help can be had from such measures as one-handed knife and fork combined, non-slip mats and suction-foot eggcup for the hemiplegic patient and cutlery with modified handles for arthritic patients. The importance of the nurse's contribution to walking retraining has already been stressed. It is essential that the nurse is fully conversant with the techniques used. In general, she needs to do all she can to encourage patients to be as active as they can and to make the ward a lively and stimulating place.

The Social Worker

The social worker needs to be involved in the general management and assessment of the patient's social problems from the earliest possible stage. Social problems need to be tackled early otherwise delays when the patient is ready to leave hospital are likely to be the cause of considerable demoralisation. Throughout the hospital stay, the social worker is able to give great support and encouragement to the patient and to help minimise anxieties about the uncertainties of the future by discussing realistic plans with him. She will be intimately involved in the discharge arrangements, arranging the necessary social services for example.

The Doctor

It is not enough for the doctor to make the necessary physical and mental assessments of the patient and then hand over responsibility for rehabilitation to other members of the rehabilitation staff. It is essential that he assumes a coordinating role if the staff are truly to function as a rehabilitation *team*. He is the person best able to ensure effective communication between the team members, ward rounds at which other members of the team are present being a particularly fruitful opportunity. He can do much to encourage different disciplines to work in close collaboration rather than in isolation or at cross purposes for the benefit of his elderly patients. He alone is able to make certain that rehabilitation starts at the earliest possible moment and is not something that happens almost as an after thought when medical treatment is completed. Finally his interest, enthusiasm and leadership are crucial to the morale of the rehabilitation team and thus to the quality of rehabilitation which can be achieved because of the central position of prestige which the doctor tends to have accorded to him in his hospital work.

The general practitioner also needs to be "rehabilitation minded" and have a working knowledge of the potential benefits of hospital rehabilitation of the elderly. He can then refer patients early when their prognosis is most favourable rather than leave matters until a crisis situation forces admission, by which time treatment may be much more difficult and outcome uncertain. He can also do a great deal in preparing his patients for admission and the persuasion, encouragement and explanation he gives at home can have enormous benefits in terms of the patient's morale and motivation.

WALKING RETRAINING

Walking retraining is such a common and important part of the rehabilitation of the geriatric patient that more detailed consideration of the techniques used is justified. It is most commonly needed for immobility due to a period of enforced inactivity rather than for specific neurological or locomotor disability. Again the importance of starting rehabilitation at the earliest practicable moment needs to be re-emphasised for if it is delayed balance particularly will deteriorate rapidly so that rehabilitation becomes progressively more difficult.

The first stage in remobilisation is to get up from a chair. The feet are positioned well under the chair, that the head and trunk are bent well forwards so as to bring the centre of gravity over the feet and that the chair, apart from having arms, should not have too low a seat height. If these requirements are met, the patient can rise from the chair with very little expenditure of energy but if assistance is necessary it can be given with a hand lifting from beneath the arm. Figure 4, part 1, shows the correct technique being used to rise from a chair; from this position the patient can take hold of a walking frame, transferring a single hand to the frame initially so that the other hand which is still on the chair arm can continue to safeguard balance (part 2). The second hand can then move safely to the frame which is now advanced some eighteen inches or so (part 3). After it has been firmly planted on the ground, each foot is advanced by one step which should be fairly short as balance to the rear becomes insecure if the patient walks too far into the frame; part 4 shows the correct position at the end of

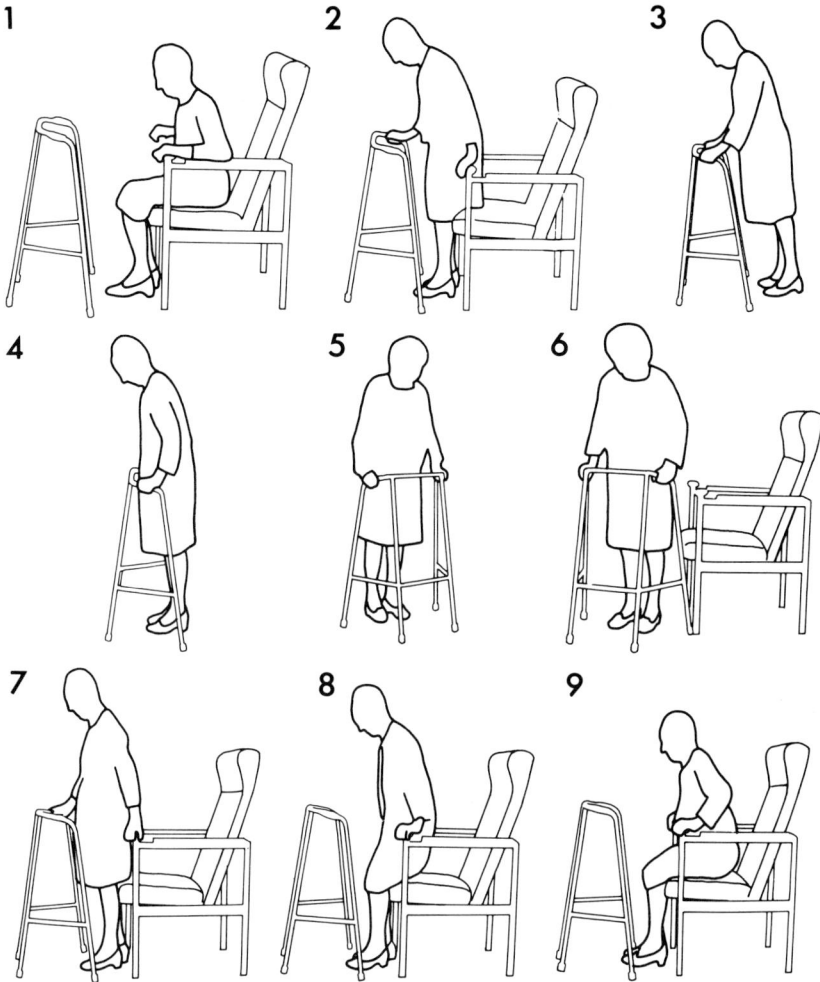

Fig. 4, parts 1-9. Correct use of the walking frame.

the two steps. It is an advantage for the patient to adopt a stooped posture and to lean quite heavily onto the frame as balance is then very secure, whereas a backward-leaning posture is unsafe. Walking now proceeds by repeating the sequence, frame—first step—second step. Simple though this sequence is, repeated instructions and corrections are commonly required by forgetful old patients. It is important that these repeated directions should be simply expressed and that if they are given by different individuals at different times that they remain consistent so as not to make confusion worse confounded. Indeed simplicity, repetition and consistency are the fundamentals of geriatric rehabilitation.

Having walked around, the patient now needs to return safely to his chair. Accidents involving the elderly who are undergoing walking retraining principally occur at the critical stages of getting up or sitting down, just as take-off and landing are the most hazardous aspects of flying. It is vital that the correct sequences are thoroughly inculcated therefore. The essential points in regaining the sitting position are that the patient must walk right up to the chair (part 6 of Fig. 4), then cautiously angle round with the frame until the calves are in contact with the front edge of the chair (part 7) and only then transfer the hands one at a time as he did in getting up (parts 7 and 8). He can now sit safely by lowering himself whilst keeping well bent forwards using the arms to maintain balance and control the rate. Part 9 of Fig 4 shows this final stage which closely mirrors the technique used in rising from the chair.

If additional help is required in walking with the frame it is given by one or two people supporting the patient from the sides, using an arm lifting from beneath the patient's arm. Most patients rapidly gain confidence and mobility using the walking frame and easily graduate to walking with a stick or without any aids as their balance and strength are regained. Other patients who are more disabled may have to continue to use a frame but this level of activity can often be adequate to allow their return home, although they may in consequence be effectively housebound.

The frame is the usually preferred aid in walking retraining. It is particularly suitable for the elderly because of its great stability and the confidence and security which this engenders. Some patients cannot use a frame however. Hemiplegics with only one effective hand-grip are obliged to rely on a tripod or quadruped stick. Getting up and walking follow very similar lines except that only one hand is available for use, but these one handed aids give far less stability and help than the frame. Parkinsonian patients may also have great difficulty in using the ordinary frame because of its stop-start technique and may do better with a wheeled frame which allows a more continuous gait pattern.

PREPARING FOR DISCHARGE

A brief home visit accompanied by the occupational therapist or physiotherapist can be very useful, particularly if hospital stay has been a long one. It can help to reassure the patient that discharge really is a serious proposition and at the same time A.D.L. can be checked in the home setting and any remaining difficulties identified so that they can be overcome by further treatment. If the patient lives with others a weekend at home may be valuable but it may be wise to prepare for this by having the friends or relatives concerned to visit the hospital first so that they can see what the patient can and cannot do and how he should be helped. With this precaution, weekend trial discharges can be most useful in reassuring both parties and in identifying any residual areas of difficulty.

Even when patients have been in hospital only for brief periods it is still important that those who support them at home gain a clear idea of their capabilities either by talking to staff or by coming to the ward or rehabilitation department to see for themselves. Over-protective relatives are commonly encountered and may need considerable re-education by members of the rehabilitation staff if they are not to erode the patient's independence after discharge by underestimating his abilities and by inappropriate handling.

9

Nursing Care

The nurse's role in dealing with elderly patients has many points of difference of emphasis and these will be outlined. Practical details of geriatric nursing techniques will not be described as there are excellent accounts available (see further reading list).

THE NURSE AND HER ELDERLY PATIENT

Elderly patients are characterised by their helplessness and frailty and by the high incidence of mental disturbance. They are particularly likely to become increasingly dependent if nurses adopt too custodial an approach. The nurse must therefore constantly bear the patient's rehabilitation needs in mind, encouraging the patient to do everything he can for himself and remembering that to do such things for him, whether out of misplaced kindness or merely to save time, can only result in the further erosion of his independence and confidence. In addition, the nurse has to learn to think for her patient because confusion and apathy so often result in failure to make his needs known or to look after his own safety.

THINKING FOR THE PATIENT

An important example of the need for the nurse to think for her elderly patient is the maintenance of adequate fluid intake. Ill old people are very likely to neglect to drink sufficiently. Thirst seems to be less efficient as a safeguard but, even when they are thirsty, frail and immobile patients may be incapable of getting a drink for themselves even though a water jug is at hand and may fail to ask for help. Some may even curb their intake of fluids quite deliberately because of the fear of being incontinent of urine. Dehydration can readily occur unless the nurse is vigilant and persuades and helps the patient to drink. The consequences of dehydration may be severe, uraemia readily developing in view of the generally poor renal function in the aged.

Another case is that of the drug round where many elderly patients cannot be relied on to take the tablets that the nurse has given to them. For reasons best known to themselves and perhaps because they often find tablet swallowing difficult and uncomfortable, patients may become masters of deception. The pill goes in the mouth all right and so does the flushing draught of water and an affirmative answer is given to the nurse's enquiry "has it gone down". But as soon as she moves on, the offending pill is surreptitiously removed and cunningly disposed of in bed, flower vase or pocket. The need for close supervision to ensure that tablets are swallowed means that medicine rounds are very time-consuming indeed. Doctors need to realise this and can save a lot of time for the trained nurses involved if they make sure that all the tablets they prescribe are really necessary and if they consider fluid preparations as alternatives.

ACCEPTANCE OF REASONABLE RISKS

The geriatric nurse needs to accept reasonable risks for her patients. Whilst there is a clear need to prevent unnecessary accidents, over-caution must be avoided if patients are not to be made into dependent invalids. Patients must be allowed to attempt to walk and do other things by themselves even though this involves some small element of risk for only by these attempts can they regain their confidence and independence. Over-protective attitudes summed up by such admonitions as "don't walk on your own or you'll fall" can totally demoralise patients and effectively frustrate their rehabilitation. Excessive use of cot-sides at night is another over-protective practice which can have bad psychological effects on patients. Similarly, the nurse looking after confused wandering patients should try to help them by finding activities which interest them and help them to retain or regain orientation. Merely trying to prevent wandering by physical restraint out of a misguided over-emphasis of physical safety often gives rise to greater restlessness or even truculence.

REST IN BED

The importance of minimising bed rest in the management of elderly patients has already been stressed. Patients are usually up for at least part of the day and only the very ill stay in bed completely. However there are some old people who love to stay in bed and are capable of going to some lengths to get their own way. The nurse will need to recognise these "artful dodgers" and distinguish them from patients who are genuinely indisposed so as to justify a day in bed.

The hospital day can be a long one and many patients will benefit from a short nap during the day. A time to lie on top of the bed and take a rest can often be set aside after lunch without interfering with rehabilitation or medical and nursing activities.

NURSING THE HELPLESS PATIENT

Geriatric patients include many whose dependency is high. Nursing care of such heavy immobile patients can be helped considerably by such aids as hoists, wheelchairs, sanitary chairs and adjustable height beds. Bathing often poses problems and bathrooms need to be sufficiently large and with the bath free-standing to allow nurses to help patients more readily. Bath aids such as bath seats and grab rails are a help, whilst hoists such as the Ambulift which can take the patient from his bed right to the bath and lower him in are of enormous value. Showers or special baths such as the Medic bath may provide useful alternatives.

INCONTINENCE

Incontinence of urine is a major problem in geriatrics, affecting something like a quarter to a half of patients who are admitted. It may have many causes but important general factors are immobility, severe illness and mental impairment.

The common situation is that of the "irritable bladder" where bladder capacity is small and is emptied frequently and incompletely. It is often associated with dementia or diffuse cerebral damage and represents a diminution of the cerebral inhibitory control of the bladder. Infection is also commonly a complicating factor. Patients experience frequency and urgency and when, as is so often the case, mobility is poor, incontinence results because the bladder and not the patient wins the race against time. Other patients may get no warning of micturition at all and this is particularly the case when there is severe dementia or central nervous system damage.

However, in most patients, cerebral inhibitory control is reduced rather than lost so that much can be done to help them to regain continence. Psychological factors are important; anxiety will usually make matters worse so that too much attention focused on the patient's failures, particularly if accompanied by expressions of irritation or blame, will prove to be detrimental. On the other hand too complacent an attitude is unhelpful and what is needed is to put value on continence, give positive encouragement to its achievement but to praise success rather than dwell unduly on failure or in any way penalise it. The adequacy of toilet accommodation has considerable relevance in winning back continence. It is a great help to have generous toilet provision on wards and that the toilets are well sited for easy access, well heated in the winter and adequately lit at night so that there are no disincentives to their use by the patients.

Treatment of infection is of great importance and when successful may lead to the return of continence. Improvement in mobility resulting from rehabilitation may also of itself improve incontinence.

Intelligent patients may learn to cope with their irritable bladder by making frequent visits to the toilet so as to forestall their frequency and urgency. Confused patients may benefit similarly if such a regime is organised for them and they are persuaded to empty the bladder at regular intervals. To arrive at the most suitable regime, it is very useful to chart the patient's pattern of incontinence first. This can indicate the appropriate frequency and timing of prompts to empty the bladder. Many are particularly likely to be incontinent when in bed and particularly first thing in the morning and this pattern may dictate the need for a toilet call during the night or immediately on waking in the morning.

Atropine-like drugs are sometimes used in an attempt to control the irritable bladder but are generally disappointing in practice and also not without troublesome side-effects.

Less commonly, incontinence is associated with an atonic bladder. Here the bladder is chronically over-filled and overflows with only partial emptying. The atonic bladder may occur in association with obstructive lesions such as prostatic enlargement or secondary to faecal impaction. Occasionally it is due to neurological disease resulting in denervation of the bladder. In many patients, especially in females, there may be no clear cause. The atonic bladder may result in dribbling incontinence but in other patients intermittent incontinence of large volumes of urine may occur.

Continence may be regained if obstructive lesions can be dealt with successfully. In other cases bladder retraining may be attempted by indwelling catheterisation and intermittent drainage for a period of some days. This may lead to the regaining of bladder tone and continence.

Stress incontinence is another possibility and is most often seen in elderly women with prolapse or with pelvic floor damage due to child-bearing. Incontinence occurs on coughing, straining or on first standing up. Sometimes surgical repair operations may be possible but in frail old patients such intervention may not always be practicable.

Incontinence can be improved or controlled in many patients but in some, particularly those with significant degrees of dementia, this is not possible. Even for the intractably incontinent there are many ways to make management easier, for example plastic incontinence pants, penile clamps, condom drainage and other male incontience appliances, the use of portable urinals and incontinence pads. Permanent catheterisation is to be regarded very much as a last resort which may, however, prove to be unavoidable. It carries very serious risks of the development of urinary infection and the more demented patients often fail to tolerate the catheter and quite often pull it out with the balloon still inflated and may occasion considerable urethral trauma to themselves. Even temporary catheterisation should be undertaken only if there are pressing reasons because of the danger of infection but also because the catheter and drainage bag can be a great hinderance to rehabilitation as well as detrimental to the patient's dignity and morale. The effects of the catheter and drainage bag on mobility can indeed be compared to those of the prisoner's ball and chain in days of old!

REGULATION OF THE BOWELS

The bowels are a cause of great concern to their elderly owners. Nurses are likely to receive many requests for assistance in the relief of constipation but the usual state of affairs in the elderly is that of faecal impaction. The rectum becomes over-full with a mass of faeces which the patient cannot expel unaided. Rectal examination must be freely used to recognise this situation for if purgatives are used for faecal impaction, the results are often little short of disastrous, their effect being to produce considerable abdominal pain and discomfort and the passage of fluid stool around the impacted mass which the patient remains incapable of passing. This "spurious diarrhoea" often produces faecal incontinence. The use of oral liquid paraffin is also to be avoided as this will merely seep past the obstructing mass and result in soiling. Added to this there is a small but serious risk of aspiration of paraffin into the lungs which can produce an intractable chemical pneumonia.

Impaction instead needs to be dealt with from below and major impaction usually calls for manual removal in the first instance. Enemas have an important role and may need to be repeated daily many times in order to clear the lower bowel completely for faecal masses may fill almost the whole of the colon. Plain water, soap and water or phosphate enemas are most often used but if large volumes cannot be retained, small volume enemas such as olive oil retention enemas are of value. Locally active suppositories such as glycerine suppositories or beogex suppositories given regularly are also very helpful, particularly in milder cases or to follow on from manual removal or enemas. Suppositories containing purgatives which are absorbed systemically, such as dulcolax suppositories, should be avoided as they suffer from all the possible drawbacks of oral purgation. When the stools are very hard, faecal softeners taken orally may be of minor assistance; these are wetting agents which help the rehydration of inspissated faeces.

Prevention of further episodes of faecal impaction requires efforts to increase the bulk content of the diet. Most old people eat a diet that contains little residue and this results in a small volume of very hard faeces which are difficult to move through the large bowel and to expel. Increased residue gives a far larger volume of softer faeces which the large gut peristaltic and emptying movements can act upon far more efficiently. Bran is a convenient way to add residue to the diet and it can be added to breakfast cereals, soups, cakes and other foods without making these unpalatable. The patient can also be encouraged to eat more of the bulk-providing foods such as fruits and vegetables and to use brown rather than white bread. Such measures are to be preferred to the use of pharmacological bulk preparations such as methyl cellulose or isogel.

PRESSURE SORES

Because of their heavy dependency and frailty, the elderly are particularly at risk regarding the development of pressure sores and nurses must take great care to prevent these as they can have such adverse effects on the patient's progress or indeed survival. Pressure sores are of two types, superficial and deep.

Superficial Pressure Sores

These are the less serious of the two types and are typically due to abrasion of the skin such as can result by dragging the patient along the bed instead of lifting him cleanly or by the semi-recumbent patient sliding down the bed because of inadequate support. Abrasion is particularly likely to occur when the skin is soggy or inflamed so that urinary incontinence is an important adverse factor especially as neglected urinary soiling can produce a chemical inflammation of the skin due to the ammonia resulting from bacterial breakdown of urea. Cleanliness, keeping the patient dry and avoiding incorrect handling and unsuitable positioning, which can allow sliding, are the main preventive measures. Skin care should involve simple washing and careful drying and talc powdering may have some value because of its dry lubricant properties. Irritant applications such as spirit or even over-generous use of soap are detrimental. The value of skin applications such as zinc cream or silicone creams or sprays is not proven although they are extensively used.

When superficial sores have occurred, they should be treated by cleaning with a non-irritant lotion such as eusol and then, where possible, left dry. Where covering is necessary non-stick nylon dressings are suitable but tulle gras, which tends to macerate the skin, is best avoided. More complicated local applications and particularly antibiotic creams or sprays are also unnecessary and potentially dangerous as they may lead to sensitivity reactions.

Deep Pressure Sores

The deep sore is a far more serious lesion which develops when tissues overlying a bony structure are compressed against it for a sufficient length of time. The resulting compression prevents blood flow through the tissue and leads to ischaemic necrosis. Subcutaneous tissues, especially muscle, are more vulnerable than the skin itself so that irreparable damage may have occurred beneath the surface for some days before the skin becomes obviously non-viable at the surface. The deep part of the sore may also be more extensive and so result in extensive undermining such as is often seen in sacral sores. The commonest sites for deep pressure sores are over the sacrum, femoral trochanters, heels and external malleoli of the ankles. Ischial sores are not common except where patients have been nursed in a chair for long periods. However deep sores can occur over any bony point where the soft tissues can be compressed.

A healthy person does not develop pressure sores because ischaemia produces the warning of discomfort and leads to relieving movement so that even in sleep movement is frequent throughout the night. Ill patients become vulnerable when unconsciousness, drowsiness or neurological disease interfere with the appreciation of pain and discomfort or when frailty or locomotor or neurological disease make movement difficult or impossible. Over-sedation is thus a dangerous adverse factor. In addition it seems that the general condition of the patient may also make the development of sores more likely. Certainly hypotension could be expected to favour their development but other factors such as fever, anaemia, dehydration and poor nutrition are also believed to be relevant.

Prevention of deep pressure sores thus involves the avoidance of unrelieved pressure on the vulnerable area and also calls for effective recognition of the patients who are at risk so that preventive efforts can be most usefully deployed. As has been indicated, those most at risk are the very ill, the drowsy or unconscious and the immobile.

The cornerstone of prevention is two-hourly turning of patients, which if consistently applied to those at risk will virtually abolish bedsores. However the practicality of applying two-hourly turning to more than a very few selected patients in view of ward staffing levels outside such special units as paraplegia centres means that great selection and use of alternatives is forced upon nurses.

Large cell ripple matresses have been shown to be of definite value but supplement rather than replace turning regimes. Caution is also required as the machines can easily be accidentally unplugged or switched off or the air tubes disconnected so that the patient is left totally unprotected. Water beds are also believed to have a preventive value but are not widely used because of their practical difficulties.

The patient's position in bed is of importance. In this respect, lying flat in bed is quite good because it spreads weight over the whole body. Sitting in the semi-recumbent posture is particularly bad because it concentrates weight on the buttocks, sacrum and heels and the tendency to slide down adds considerable shearing force. Heel sores are a particular problem and may occur in patients who are up and walking by day but have difficulty moving the legs in bed when the feet are trapped by sheets that are tucked in too tightly. Patients with fracture, arthritis or parkinsonism are particularly at risk and such vulnerable patients should have a bed-cradle to take the weight of the bed clothes and in general nurses should acquire the habit of tucking bedclothes in more loosely at the foot of the bed.

The prevention of pressure sores has developed its own mythology and the true value of many measures such as lying on sheepskins, wearing of heelpads or sheepskin bootees, plastic foam or inflatable rings, special pillows and special skin creams and sprays is conjectural and dubious. Such measures may be detrimental in as much as they may detract from the fullest application of other measures which are of proven value.

The established deep sore will only heal once all the necrotic slough has gone so that active debridement is of value. Simple applications such as eusol or eusol and paraffin are to be preferred to the many esoteric recipes that claim their enthusiastic devotees such as applications of honey, marmite and much else that owes more to the larder than the pharmacy. The general condition of the patient certainly has a powerful effect on the healing of his sores and these may get worse or better as his illness waxes or wanes. Adequate diet is important and many patients with large sores may develop considerable hypo-albuminaemia and anaemia which may call for additional protein, haematinics or even transfusion. Anabolic steroids are of no value. Antibiotic therapy may occasionally be indicated, as when cellulitis develops around a sore, but has no part in the treatment of the uncomplicated pressure sore. Large sores may sometimes benefit from surgical intervention such as grafting or the rotation of skin flaps when the patient's general condition makes this a justifiable course.

The deep pressure sore represents a major disaster which has marked effects on the prognosis of the patient. Large sores have an enormously debilitating effect and are often the last straw leading to the patient's further deterioration and death. Even when not life threatening, sores heal slowly, often taking many months and so may delay or slow the rehabilitation of the patient. Rehabilitation may well be unsuccessful because of the pain, debility and demoralising effects of the long time in hospital so that a patient who might otherwise have returned home needs permanent long-stay care in hospital instead. Prevention of pressure sores thus has enormous practical importance. Experience shows that the majority of sores develop during the first week or two in hospital; perhaps because it takes time for nurses to fully recognise the needs of the patients. Identification of the patient at risk therefore needs to be prompt so that effective preventive measures can be fully mobilised during the most vulnerable period.

Further Reading
Irvine, R E, Bagnall, M K & Smith, B J (1978) The older patient, 3rd edition, English Universities Press, London.
Norton, D, McLaren, R & Exton-Smith, A N (1962) An investigation of geriatric nursing problems in hospital, The National Corporation for the Care of Old People, London.

10

Care of the Irremediable Patient

LONG-STAY PATIENTS

A small proportion of the patients admitted to a geriatric department will, despite the fullest application of medical treatment and attempts at rehabilitation, fail to make a sufficient improvement to allow their return to the community and need care in hospital for the rest of their life. Geriatric departments also acquire other patients who need long-stay care from other hospital departments by transfer, although commonly they will be admitted to an active ward in the first instance to make quite certain that no therapeutic opportunities are overlooked. This is a most important safeguard for all patients who enter a long-stay ward and in most cases they will have been in hospital for at least several weeks before they are transferred there. As already noted, long-stay wards are often situated in small peripheral hospitals without full district general hospital facilities emphasising the necessity for full investigation and assessment before patients go there.

Most of the patients in long-stay accommodation are females, usually only about a fifth are males. The age distribution differs little from that of all patients admitted to the department. The overwhelming majority of the patients will be confused and incontinent and will have considerable physical disabilities and poor mobility. Many have cerebro-vascular disease, some being hemiplegics who have major intellectual loss and so could not be successfully rehabilitated, others arteriosclerotic dementia patients with considerable physical disability. Dysphasia, poor vision and deafness are common complicating disabilities. Only a small minority of the long-stay population are patients with a well-preserved mental state and most of these are patients with very gross disabilities such as advanced rheumatoid arthritis.

Those who become long-stay patients are more likely to have had multiple previous admissions to hospital, to have been socially isolated or to have been admitted from an old people's home. The majority of long-stay patients are ultimately destined to die in hospital though a minority are eventually discharged. Discharge is far more likely to be to an old people's home rather than the patient's home, however.

LONG-STAY CARE

Most long-stay care of elderly patients takes place in designated long-stay wards as almost all departments of geriatric medicine practice some form of progressive patient care based on admission, rehabilitation and long-stay wards. Long-stay wards are commonly situated in small local hospitals rather than in the main district general hospital. Even though long-stay patients may only account for some 5% or so of all the patients admitted to a department of geriatric medicine, they may occupy half or more of all the beds. Long-stay care is thus a very important part of hospital provision for old people. Its usual physical separation from the acute medical and rehabilitation aspects of the work of a department of geriatric medicine has potential dangers but also many important advantages.

Separate long-stay wards, and most particularly those sited in specifically long-stay hospitals, may become professionally isolated and may lag behind in terms of physical upgrading in consequence. These possibilities need to be guarded against. The potential advantages are, in any case, far greater for there is the chance to create a total pattern of care which is entirely appropriate to the needs of long-stay patients. Certainly these needs are often poorly met in admission and rehabilitation wards. They are organised on a predominantly medical model which is largely inappropriate.

Ordinary rehabilitation has largely physical aims, particularly geared to the patient's discharge home. Achievement of mobility, continence and competence in relevant activities of daily living are major aims. These goals may be impossible or irrelevant to the long-stay patient. Instead, our aims must be to preserve the individual's personality against the insidious pressures of institutionalisation with its resultant features of apathy, misery and passivity. The patient needs to find purpose in his remaining life, particularly now that prospects of discharge no longer provide realistic motivation. Staff need to develop a positive yet honest approach, not allowing obvious disabilities to blind them to the residual abilities of the patient which can be developed and utilised.

Half-hearted continuation of rehabilitation programmes with physical goals which are no longer realistic is likely to be harmful rather than beneficial and, perhaps too frequently, "diversional therapy" may be a euphemism for unimaginative repetitive activities which bore rather than stimulate. Instead of ill-conceived "therapy" we need to create opporutnities for individual patients to make their own decisions, to enjoy meaningful work, to learn and to interact socially. There is great scope for imagination and innovation so that the best possible use can be made of local educational, recreational, professional and voluntary resources and so that relatives and friends can play a full part.

The Nursing Role

Multidisciplinary collaboration is as important in long-stay care as in any aspect of geriatric work but nursing staff have a key part to play. Long-stay patients have a high degree of nursing dependency so that their care is physically exacting. Yet good long-stay units usually have no difficulty in recruiting and retaining nursing staff. Perhaps this is because of the special challenges of long-stay care. In particular, many nurses achieve great satisfaction from the close and sustained relationships with their patients and from the recognition of the pre-eminence of the nursing role in this sphere. Only they can create the right home-like atmosphere and are best placed to encourage visiting, group activities, weekend leave arrangements where these are practicable, outings, diversional therapy and social activities involving local residents and voluntary organisations. The aim is to create a relaxed atmosphere with the maximum of human interest and a minimum of starchiness, rules and regimentation. Wherever possible patients are up and dressed and encouraged to live as full a life as they can.

The incidence of pressure sores is usually extremely low in long-stay units because of the skill and experience of the staff but also because, although the patients are heavily disabled, their condition is stable and their needs well recognised so that adequate preventive measures are taken.

MEDICAL ASPECTS OF LONG-STAY CARE

Medical treatment must be tailored to the special features of long-stay patients. When patients are slowly and inevitably deteriorating it is essential to temper excessive therapeutic zeal. Thus resuscitation rarely has a place and in many instances it may be more fitting to withold antibiotics for pneumonia, the old man's friend, when this ushers in a peaceful release from a long and trying illness. Quality of life and not its length should be the prime concern and symptomatic treatment, for example with opiates for pain, should not be denied when the patient's life would be made more bearable even at the cost of some risk to its duration. Despite the prevalence of dementia and confusion, the staff of a good long-stay unit should rely very little on the use of night sedation and tranquillisers. A tolerant and resourceful nursing staff rarely need to use them and so avoid the problems of hangover, apathy, drowsiness and increased incontinence and immobility that they inevitably produce.

Long-stay care is not primarily medical: we have already noted the far greater importance of the nursing contribution. However, medical staff still have an important part to play. Medical leadership is often an important aspect of the dynamics of a successful multidisciplinary team and doctors need to contribute their share of new ideas along with all the other professional groups forming the team. They can give important practical, moral and political support to innovation.

Their purely medical input is relatively limited. Patients transferred to long-stay care will already have been fully investigated and diagnosed and are usually clinically stable. Medical care is mainly concerned with episodes of intercurrent illness. However the medical staff need to keep a careful watch for patients who may make an unexpected late recovery which re-opens the possibility of discharge and makes transfer back to a rehabilitation ward appropriate. Such late recoveries are not particularly uncommon for the stimulating environment of a good long-stay unit may encourage a new flowering of motivation when earlier lack of it had precluded successful rehabilitation.

TERMINAL CARE

Something like half of all deaths over 65 now take place in hospitals and geriatric departments carry a considerable part of this load. Many deaths occur soon after admission during the phase of active treatment of patients with severe illness or represent sudden and perhaps unexpected deaths such as those due to pulmonary embolism or a rapidly overwhelming pneumonia.

A substantial number of deaths occur however in patients who have serious disease which is considered irremediable and likely to lead to early death. It is these patients requiring terminal care who present particular problems in comparison with the foregoing groups although a large number of deaths of any type can have demoralising effects on staff, especially on nurses in the early part of their training.

Malignant disease is a common cause of illness calling for terminal care. Accurate diagnosis and prognosis is essential, previously made diagnoses should not be accepted uncritically if therapeutic opportunities are not to be missed. In particular the possibility of the development of a second disease accounting for the present deterioration which is treatable must be remembered. It is easy to assume that the marked deterioration in a patient who had a gastrectomy for carcinoma of stomach some time before is due to the primary disease but his pains could be due to the development of osteomalacia or his anaemia, weight loss and malaise to pernicious anaemia as complications of gastrectomy. Treatment may also be still possible despite advanced metastatic disease, as for example in the hormonal treatment of carcinoma of prostate or breast which can result in useful remissions.

ATTITUDES TO DEATH

The attitudes towards death of staff, patients and the community at large have a considerable bearing on terminal care. Thus doctors and nurses are at risk of being so geared to the philosophy of cure that death is regarded as a humiliating failure. Further they are not immune to the shortcomings of the members of the community at large who regard death as an unmentionable subject occasioning fear and embarassment. Staff with such emotional attitudes to death will be ill equiped to give the best possible care to dying patients. They may try to avoid having to deal with them or when obliged to do so may be unable to accept their therapeutic limitations and so persist in unrealistic efforts to cure which may salve their own consciences but which are grossly unfair to the patient.

Psychological Support

It has been truly said that "only those who have come to terms with the idea of their own dying can cope with the needs of terminal patients" (Lancet editorial, 1971) and enlightened staff can play a most helpful role in assisting dying patients and their relatives to deal with their emotional reactions to the situation. Whilst many old people lapse into a state of confusion, clouding of consciousness or coma as death approaches, others remain mentally clear and may need this psychological understanding and support. Many become slowly but increasingly aware of the likelihood or certainty of their own imminent death and may indeed have powerful premonition of it.

Many old people meet their approaching death with exemplary calmness and dignity and indeed often take the view that they have had "a good innings" so that after a taxing illness they see death as a friend and not an enemy. It is other patients who have less satisfactory reactions who require help. Anxiety calls for sympathetic support which can give far more help than tranquillisers or sedatives. Staff need particular understanding and forbearance when the patient projects his emotion onto them in the form of aggressive, over-clinging, critical or paranoid behaviour. Depression is another important reaction and may be sufficiently severe to present a suicide risk or to call for specific treatment which may give valuable relief even in severely ill patients.

Patients' religious beliefs can be a powerful sustaining influence during terminal illness and the hospital chaplain or the patient's own minister can give most useful support.

Whether to Tell

Whether or not the terminal patient should be told his true prognosis is a question which is the subject of endless debate. There can be no rule of thumb for one must be guided by the patient himself and be prepared for frank discussion if this is appropriate.

In fact, many patients do put two and two together and have reasonably certain knowledge of their likely fate. Some may gently fish for confirmation and should be led on to as full a discussion as they appear to wish. It is pointless to deny the possibility of death for this can only give the most fleeting reassurance at best and needlessly destroys the patient's trust in his attendants. Other patients prefer to keep their suspicions to themselves and their reticence should be respected. Others again prefer to play games of transparent self deception, denying the seriousness of the situation, and staff can usually join in the game on the patient's terms in the full knowledge that both sides know it is a game which is not fooling anyone.

It is of course essential that next of kin are informed of the true prognosis and have the opportunity for full discussion. Unfortunately if the relative does know and the patient doesn't there can sometimes be an erosion of their relationship with each other because of the dishonesties this situation makes necessary. This may often give rise to sufficient problems to tip the balance in favour of telling the patient the full facts.

Symptomatic Treatment

Successful terminal care also calls for effective management of distressing symptoms. Pain can almost always be satisfactorily controlled and the best policy is to give analgesics of sufficient potency early enough and generously enough so that the patient's confidence in the effectiveness of pain relief is firmly established and maintained. Potent analgesics such as morphine or heroin should not be held back because of irrelevant fears of their addictive properties and it is essential that patients are not given analgesia grudgingly and half-heartedly so that their confidence in pain relief is shattered for it has been found that such patients are likely to need far more analgesia later. Heroin is a particularly valuable drug as it has euphoriant as well as powerful analgesic effects and causes far less drowsiness and nausea than other opiates. It is unstable in aqueous solution so that if used in a "Brompton Mixture" this needs to be freshly prepared.

Nausea and vomiting are particularly distressing symptoms but fortunately can usually be fairly well controlled by phenothiazines such as intramuscular promazine. More difficult symptoms to alleviate are dyspnoea, dysphagia, itching and the general malaise and lassitude of severe illness.

Surgical palliation always calls for careful appraisal and should only be undertaken in terminal illness when it is clear that anticipated benefits to the patient outweigh the unpleasantness of the treatment and that in preserving the patient from one unpleasantness we do not lay him open to a worse one to follow. An example of this is the now totally discredited operation of gastrostomy in malignant oesophageal obstruction. This allowed the patient to be fed and hydrated but left him to drown in his own saliva which he remained unable to swallow.

General Policies

The general policies of terminal care can be summed up in the phrase "death with dignity". Technical medicine must not be allowed to run out of hand and no patient with terminal illness should die with tubes in every available orifice. Cicely Saunders (1973), who has made such enormous contributions in the field of terminal care, sums this up cogently

> it is far better to have a cup of tea on your last day than drips and tubes in every direction. And I think this cup of tea comes best from someone who has compassion, understanding and practicality—someone who does add heart to skill and has a sense of meaning and assurance of another dimension of life. We should never impose our own beliefs and our own feelings of meaning on to another person, but I am quite sure we could help to produce a climate in which the

patients can find their own meanings, and can find the quietness and dignity of death as it can be when it is a person not the apparatus around that is the centre of attention.

Orientation must shift from cure to care and so elaborate and taxing dressings of wounds or pressure sores should yield to the minimum procedure needed for the patient's comfort. Inessential treatments and routines should be withdrawn if this will assist the patient to find comfort and rest. New treatment such as antibiotics for an episode of infection is only justifiable if it is likely to improve the quality of the terminal patient's remaining life. Attempts to prolong dying or to resuscitate when death does occur can have no justification whatsoever.

When and Where

One problem of terminal care is the patient who is admitted at too early a stage, perhaps because his general practitioner has been overawed by the seriousness of the diagnosis and has taken an unduly pessimistic view of the prognosis.

In general it is wise for such patients to be discharged home again quickly with the undertaking that they can be readmitted without delay when the true need finally arises. The patient may then enjoy a period of some weeks or even months in his own home before the last short phase of his illness for which he needs full hospital care. He avoids a long and demoralising stay in hospital during which he might very likely become upset or disgruntled by the lack of active therapy.

Geriatric departments are sometimes asked to accept younger patients for terminal care. I believe it to be entirely inappropriate for such patients to be nursed in geriatric wards. Patient and relatives tend to be upset by the nature of the ward and it seems far more fitting that their care should be provided either in the general hospital department which has dealt with them earlier or in a specialised terminal care unit.

In the geriatric ward, as a terminal patient nears death, nursing staff need to decide where in the ward nursing care is best provided. Single rooms are often utilised so that distress to other patients may be minimised and to allow quiet and more ready visiting by his relatives for the patient. However the single room may isolate the patient unduly so that he lacks the human company and support that are so important as death draws near. Furthermore, if the same room or bed is commonly used for this purpose it may gain a well-recognised reputation with adverse effects on patient morale.

The Death

In the terminal care situation the diagnosis of death seldom presents particular difficulties but, as indeed for any hospital death, it is important that this remains a medical responsibility and is not delegated to nursing staff. When there are difficulties, ophthalmoscopy and the recognition of "trucking", the breaking up into segments of the column of blood in the retinal vessels, is a clear-cut sign which develops rapidly.

Removal of the body from the ward after death can often be carried out in a furtive and hurried manner with much drawing of curtains and evasiveness and uneasiness if other patients ask questions. It is clearly better for all concerned if the death on the ward can be handled in a dignified and solemn way but with greater openness and honesty. When other patients ask after the deceased patient they need to be told the truth and not fobbed off with falsehoods such as "oh, she's been transferred to another ward".

Medical and nursing staff often need to give psychological support and also practical guidance as to the formalities to the bereaved relatives. They may also need to mobilise continuing support especially for an elderly bereaved spouse. Many studies have shown the great vulnerability to develop depression and social isolation in this situation and the general practitioner and community social workers may be key sources of help.

Further Reading

British Geriatrics Society and Royal College of Nursing of the United Kingdom (1978) Improving geriatric care in hospital, Royal College of Nursing, London.
Hodkinson, I & Hodkinson, H M (1981) The long-stay patient, Gerontology, in press.
Saunders, C (1959) Care of the dying, Macmillan, London.
Twycross, R G (1975) The dying patient, Christian Medical Fellowship, London.

11

Drug Therapy in the Elderly

In no small part, the achievements of geriatrics in terms of the improvement of the care of old people have depended on the general advances in drug therapy that have occurred in the last twenty-five years or so. It has been repeatedly demonstrated that the application of these therapies after proper diagnostic evaluation in elderly patients can give results that are fully comparable to those in other age-groups.

However, the undoubted benefits of these therapeutic advances are often marred by injudicious treatment and by the occurence of side effects and drug interactions in the elderly. For while the principles of good therapeutics are no different in old age, the many pitfalls of careless prescribing can be most strikingly illustrated in considering the treatment of the elderly.

DRUG SIDE EFFECTS

The frequency of drug side effects rises with age as well as with the number of drugs prescribed. There are a number of reasons why the elderly are at special risk. Firstly there are changes in body composition with age. Lean body mass tends to decrease whilst there is a relative increase in body fat. This has complex effects on drug pharmocokinetics in elderly people. Drugs that are actively metabolised by the body will tend to have longer half-lives due to the reduced lean body mass which represents actively metabolising cells and overdose effects are more likely. Body water is also relatively reduced so that water soluble drugs will tend to achieve higher levels again favouring overdosage. Fat soluble drugs in contrast will have prolonged half-lives but this depot storage effect may make the drug less effective in the short term though far more likely to give cummulative overdose effects. Altered drug binding associated with the fall in albumin with age further complicates these changes in distribution of drugs leading to a variety of changes in drug half-lives and in the potential for toxic effects.

Renal function is also generally reduced in old age and more particularly in ill old people. Many drugs are excreted by the kidneys and these are far more likely to give toxic side effects in old age. Pharmokinetics of drugs also depend on the rate and extent of absorbtion but these appear to be little changed in old age.

70

Perhaps even more important than alterations in pharmacokinetics are changes in the vulnerability of organs or systems in old age. The brain in particular shows greater susceptibility so that drug-induced confusional states occur far more commonly in the old. Similarly the parkinsonian and dyskinetic side effects of phenothiazines are particularly seen in the elderly patient. Homoeostatic mechanisms are less efficient and more readily disturbed so that drug-induced hypotension or the precipitation of hypothermia are more likely. The higher prevalence of pre-symptomatic disease may also lead to such side effects as the induction of diabetes or precipitation of an attack of gout by the thiazide diuretics. Already poor skeletal mass makes the osteoporotic side effect of cortico-steroid therapy far more hazardous.

MULTIPLE THERAPY

Because diagnoses are so often multiple in old age, the temptation to indulge in multiple prescribing is particularly strong. Even worse is the careless prescription of multiple symptomatic treatments for the varied symptoms of old people in whom no proper diagnosis has been made. Multiple prescribing causes a disproportionate increase in the risks of adverse effects. One factor is that of errors in taking the prescribed drugs. Most patients will make serious errors as soon as they have to contend with more than two or three different drugs and when the patient is old, confused, apathetic, depressed or partially sighted the liability to error is clearly much greater. The commonest errors are those of omission and here one sometimes suspects the operation of the divine hand of providence and speculates as to whether survival into ripe old age is not largely due to this protective device! More serious are errors leading to overdosage, especially when potent and toxic drugs such as digitalis are involved.

Multiple prescribing may also produce dangers because of the additive effects of drugs with similar actions or of the opposed antagonistic effects of pairs of drugs given for different reasons. These however are comparatively minor problems compared to those due to drug interactions.

DRUG INTERACTIONS

Drugs given together may interact in many, often complex, ways and such interaction may result in either treatment being rendered ineffective or in serious hazards. It will suffice to consider some of the main mechanisms.

Plasma Binding Effects

Many drugs are partially bound to the plasma proteins, the bound portion being pharmacologically inactive although providing a depot of the drug, while the free drug is responsible for the drug's activity and for its toxic effects. Albumin is the chief binding protein and many weakly acidic drugs appear to share the same binding sites which have a limited capacity. Such drugs given together compete for the binding sites or starting a second drug can displace the first drug and lead to an important rise in its free concentration. Thus if a patient who is well controlled on anticoagulant therapy with warfarin is then given a drug such as aspirin or phenylbutazone, warfarin will be displaced and dangerous over-anticoagulation result. Plasma bindings effects are particularly important in the elderly because albumin levels are often very low, particularly when the subject is ill, so that the relative proportion of unbound drug is already high.

Enzyme Induction

Where drugs are metabolised by the liver, their continued administration can lead to an increase in the activity of the related microsomal enzyme systems and this may persist for some time after the drug has been stopped. The more active enzyme systems result in more rapid destruction of the drug itself which may lead to reduced therapeutic effectiveness but in addition will cause the more rapid destruction of other drugs or normal metabolites which utilise the same enzyme systems. So other drugs given subsequently may be made relatively ineffective. In the elderly there is a special risk of the enzyme inducing effects of such drugs as the barbiturates given continuously as night sedatives or anti-epiletics. This can result in increased breakdown of active vitamin D metabolites. As vitamin D intakes are often low and as synthesis depends on ultra-violet light exposure which may be much reduced in elderly disabled people, this can readily result in the development of osteomalacia.

Enzyme Inhibition

Some drugs have the opposite effect, that of reducing the activity of certain enzyme systems. An example are the mono-amine-oxidase inhibitors used as antidepressants. Amine-oxidase enzymes are important in the detoxication of many biologically active amines and the administration of these as drugs (e.g. ephedrine or amphetamines) or their ingestion as food (e.g. matured cheese) can give rise to serious toxic effects, even precipitating cerebral haemorrhage as a consequence of their pressor actions.

Interference with Absorption

Drugs may interfere with each other's absorption from the gut. For example, metallic substances such as iron salts or aluminium hydroxide may hinder the absorption of tetracycline antibiotics because of complex formation.

Digitalis and Diuretics

Digitalis intoxication is far more common when oral diuretics are being given concurrently. This is because the latter may cause potassium depletion, particularly likely in the elderly who often have a very poor dietary intake of potassium, and this enhances the activity and toxicity of digitalis.

PROBLEMS OF OVER-TREATMENT

Over-treatment occurs with regrettable frequency in elderly patients. Multiple diagnoses often lead to the prescription of multiple drugs and when these result in side effects there is a real danger that these are not recognised and that further treatment is added to deal with the new symptoms!

In prescribing for the elderly it is essential that a number of common sense rules are heeded. Treatment should never be worse than the disease. Indeed treatment should offer clear superiority over no treatment and should never be given with the vague hope that it *might* do some good or to salve the prescriber's conscience. The prescriber must accept the inherent short-comings of medicine and recognise that there is not a pill for every ill. Drug regimes should never be more complex than the patient can reliably manage and this means that the number of drugs must be kept to within a realistic minimum and that individual dosage regimes should be as simple as possible. This may often mean that even drugs which, considered in isolation, can have a good case made for their use must be omitted in view of the total circumstances and the overall priorities. Finally the decision when to stop a drug is just as important as that to start it and should be given proper consideration. All too commonly, drugs are continued for long after the need for them has passed.

Some over-treatment situations are sufficiently common to justify special consideration in the following sections.

Over-prescribing of Diuretics

A surprising number of the elderly, particularly old women, are given long-term diuretic therapy with thiazides or frusemide. Often the only initial indication was ankle oedema, the cause of which was never properly diagnosed but was commonly not cardiac failure but mechanical oedema due to arthritic knees, varicose veins or simple lack of mobility and which could better have been left untreated. Alternatively, the diuretic treatment may have been started quite properly for, say, heart failure which occurred in association with acute chest infection but is then continued long after the event and quite unneccessarily.

Such unnecessary administration of diuretics may have a variety of unwanted consequences including urinary urgency or incontinence, hypo-natraemia with associated malaise and perhaps postural hypotension and hypokalaemia which may occur despite potassium supplements and lead to apathy and weakness or contribute to digitalis toxicity if this is being given concurrently.

Anti-hypertensive Drugs

These potent drugs are prescribed for the elderly on a huge scale, often on the most flimsy basis. In many, one or a few casual blood pressure readings have been found to be high and hypertension has been diagnosed and treated. Yet my experience is that when the treatment is stopped and blood pressure regularly charted many such patients prove to have no true hypertension, although capable of the odd high reading. Even when true hypertension is present it is very doubtful if more than a tiny minority of elderly patients are likely to gain from its treatment with drugs. What is beyond doubt is that many elderly patients who are given drugs for hypertension suffer serious side effects as a consequence; geriatricians see many such cases each year and find that they do much more good by stopping such treatment than by starting it in others! The adverse effects can be grave, severe hypotension leading to a cerebro-vascular catastrophe soon after treatment has been started being the most dramatic instance. One commonly encounters patients who develop severe giddiness due to postural hypotension and who become severely incapacitated, to the extent of becoming housebound, bed-ridden or suffering serious falls or fractures, as a result of the use of these drugs and who make a gratifying recovery when they are stopped. Reserpine presents a special hazard in that it may precipitate depression quite commonly in old people.

In view of these major risks, I hold the view shared by many geriatricians that hypertension in the elderly should only be treated with drugs in a small minority of cases. It must be clear that the patient is *suffering* from undoubted diastolic hypertension or that the hypertension is of such severity that the untreated prognosis fully justifies the considerable risks of treatment. We need to be sure that the institution of treatment is likely to improve the quality of the patient's life and it is not enough that it might possibly increase its length.

Hypnotics

Hypnotics are probably the most over-prescribed drugs for all age groups and the elderly do not escape this custom. Hypnotics are a symptomatic treatment and are often given without proper consideration of the possible cause of the insomnia of which the patient complains. This may be due to any one of a wide variety of causes such as depression, anxiety, nocturia, acute confusional state, dementia, paroxysmal nocturnal dyspnoea, pain or external factors such as noise or other discomforts. The appropriate treatment may thus range widely, analgesics, antidepressants, heart failure treatment, an antibiotic for urinary infection or stopping a drug responsible for a confusional state or a diuretic giving nocturia; all these may be more appropriate than prescription of a hypnotic which may be useless or positively harmful.

Even when a hypnotic is given appropriately it is essential that it is not continued any longer than is absolutely necessary for habituation readily occurs with all hypnotics, especially barbiturates. Patients suffer withdrawl symptoms when they are stopped, a rebound excess of paradoxical (R.E.M.) sleep occurring which may be accompanied by frightening dreams. They often demand the continuation of night sedation and this is often difficult to resist so that the drug is continued indefinitely with the attendant dangers of enzyme induction effects, hangover effects leading to ataxia or falls, or the development of confusional states. In depressed patients there is the special danger of the use of night sedatives as an instrument of suicide. There is no safe hypnotic, some are merely more dangerous than others.

Failure to Stop Treatment

This has already been referred to in connection with diuretics and hypnotics. Other important examples are digitalis, a particularly hazardous drug in the elderly because of poor renal function and the increased likelihood of potassium depletion, which Dall (1970) showed could be discontinued as a maintenance treatment in three-quarters of elderly patients without detriment. Similarly, many elderly diabetics receive unnecessary treatment with the sulphonylurea oral drugs, again toxic agents with such important side effects as hypoglycaemia and hyponatraemia.

CONCLUSIONS

Drug therapy of the elderly is particularly hazardous because of poor renal function, reduced active body mass and the increased vulnerability of body systems, particularly the central nervous system. The hazards are made greater by the liability of ill old people to make mistakes in taking their prescribed drugs and by the frequency with which the elderly are subjected to multiple prescribing.

Prescribing for the elderly needs to be undertaken with particular care both in regard to starting treatment and in continuing it on a maintenance basis. The total number of drugs needs to be kept within bounds as their increase leads to errors in taking them and a disproportionate risk of adverse effects and interactions.

Treatment should be started only when it is likely to improve the patient's quality of life. Treatments of dubious benefit or marginal relevance should not be undertaken; the elderly are very unsuitable as the subjects of ill-considered, uncontrolled experiments inspired by undue therapeutic optimism.

Further Reading

Denham, M J (1978) Treatment policies, Medicine (3rd series), *1*, 24-28.

O'Malley, K, Laher, M, Cusack, B & Kelly, J G (1980) Clinical pharmacology and the elderly patient, p 1-34 in The treatment of medical problems in the elderly, Ed. Denham, M J, MTP Press, Lancaster.

12

Nutrition of the Elderly

The subject of nutrition in the elderly is one which has attracted increasing interest in recent years, particularly in view of some claims that malnutrition might be very common among the aged. At the very least these claims have stimulated a number of major surveys (D.H.S.S. 1970, 1972) which have brought some hard facts to bear in an area in which the lack of information had previously permitted excessive speculation.

INGESTION AND DIGESTION

There is little evidence that structural or functional age changes have much of an impact on the ability to eat and digest food. Although many old people are edentulous, the majority have dentures and most are capable of reasonably effective mastication. Even where masticatory ability is poor, there is little evidence that overall nutrition suffers although there may be qualitative changes; soft, easy to chew foods being selected preferentially so that carbohydrate intake may become proportionally higher.

Although atrophic gastritis becomes more common with advancing age, as do abnormalities of the small bowel mucosa, these changes do not appear to result in any significant impairment of the ability to absorb food in general, although some specific nutrients such as vitamin B_{12} may possibly suffer.

NUTRITIONAL REQUIREMENTS

True nutritional requirements of the elderly are largely a matter for speculation although this does not prevent seemingly authoritative statements of minimum requirements being issued by official bodies. Certainly, rigid application of such minima would classify many old people as being malnourished when there is no objective evidence that this is the case.

Requirements are particularly complicated by the fact that different nutrients need to be related to different factors. Thus total calorie requirements relate to overall energy expenditure, so that activity level rather than mere body size is the key factor. Thiamine is needed for carbohydrate metabolism so it too principally relates to overall energy expenditure. In contrast, many other requirements are related to aspects of body size. Protein, iron, vitamin C, folate and B_{12} needs can be best related to lean body mass and calcium and vitamin D to skeletal mass.

FALL OF FOOD INTAKE WITH AGE

Activity tends to fall with age, particularly in the higher age-groups, these changes being well reviewed by Durnin (1978). Other changes are that lean body mass and skeletal mass tend to fall in response to relative disuse but fat deposits commonly increase so that total body weight may be maintained or may indeed increase.

In response to falling energy expenditure, gross calorie intake tends to fall with age, although less steeply than is suggested by cross-sectional surveys; longitudinal studies indicating that falls are unimpressive provided that subjects remain in good health but substantial if health becomes impaired. The fall in total calorie intake is achieved by eating less food, the general evidence being that this quantitative change is accompanied by remarkably little in the way of qualitative change. As energy expenditure may decline to a far greater extent than lean body mass, this leads to a situation where nutrients whose requirements relate to the latter come to be provided less generously. The risk of deficiency of such nutrients therefore becomes greater.

DIETARY DEFICIENCIES

It has been claimed that such deficiencies are frequent in the elderly but such views are not accepted by most geriatricians nor have they been supported by wide based surveys (D.H.S.S. 1970, 1972).

Energy

Energy intakes seem to be inadequate only in the setting of physical illness. Chronic illness may give rise to prolonged low calorie intakes but otherwise quite fit old people may have dramatically reduced calorie intakes during episodes of acute illness and if these are repeated they may possibly have a considerable overall effect on the long-term average intake. It seems that it is illness that leads to poor nutrition rather than poor nutrition leading to illness.

Protein

Although protein requirements relate to lean body mass and deficiency might thus be expected, clinical evidence that it in fact occurs is very difficult to come by. Carbohydrate rich foods such as bread contain useful amounts of protein so that it is in fact very difficult to achieve a low protein intake if calorie intake is reasonably good. The decrease in lean body mass appears to be due to relative disuse leading to atrophy and not to any lack of protein in the diet. The usual recommendations regarding protein requirements in old age are probably over-generous. Fears of protein lack in the elderly have probably been much exaggerated and certainly the common practices of giving protein supplements such as casilan and various proprietary concentrated special foods to patients who are eating very little are misguided. In the absence of an adequate calorie intake the extra protein will simply be used to supply calories that could have been more appropriately supplied as carbohydrate or fat.

Iron

Iron requirements are related to body size and intakes are often rather low in the elderly because of their smaller total intake of food. Iron deficiency either as diminished iron stores, low serum iron saturation or actual iron deficiency anaemia is often found in the elderly but it is not clear whether this can fairly be ascribed to dietary deficiency as careful investigation so frequently reveals abnormal blood loss, particularly as occult bleeding from the gastrointestinal tract.

Vitamins

The question of vitamin deficiency in the elderly is a rather contentious one. Some regard such deficiencies as commonplace especially among the chronic sick in institutions. Others have failed to substantiate these findings and in particular have not been able to show improvement after treatment with vitamin supplements in such clinical signs as purpura, angular stomatitis and tongue abnormalities which had been claimed as manifestations of vitamin deficiency. Many workers have found lower blood levels of vitamins or of parameters reflecting vitamin status in elderly populations compared with younger groups. However, the interpretation of such findings is not straightforward. It cannot be assumed that such lower levels imply deficiency unless it can be shown that lack of the vitamin is responsible for an actual disturbance of function or a physical abnormality in the individual. Furthermore, the "abnormality" of such lower levels is not proved if it is demonstrated that they can be raised to "normal" levels, that is levels like those in younger subjects, by giving vitamin supplements. This could merely be an indication that levels are broadly indicative of intake and that intake is higher in the young and in no way answers the question as to whether lower levels are in any way detrimental. At best, the finding of lower levels in elderly populations can only indicate the *possibility* that vitamin deficiency may be occurring and proof must rest on clinical evidence. Undoubted clinical evidence of vitamin deficiency in the elderly is seldom found and definite examples of deficiency of vitamin A, pyridoxine, riboflavin, thiamine or nicotinic acid are considerable rarities in geriatric practice. Dietary folate deficiency is fairly common, most often occurring in the setting of physical or psychiatric illness which has resulted in poor recent food intake.

Scurvy

Scurvy, the classical manifestation of vitamin C deficiency, is seen occasionally in the elderly and is perhaps the best established nutritional deficiency to be found in the age group. Those who develop clinical scurvy typically have been eating grossly abnormal diets. They may be elderly batchelors or widowers who are particularly weak on cooking skills or those who keep too strictly and too long to restricted therapeutic diets (e.g. ulcer diets) or food faddists. Total calorie intake is usually good but the diet lacks the rich sources of vitamin C—fruit, potatoes and vegetables. What vitamin C was present may be destroyed by habitual overcooking of vegetables.

The most helpful physical signs are those of abnormal bleeding, most typically as sheet haemorrhages in the legs, bleeding into the thigh muscles, widespread ecchymoses or extensive purpura. Bleeding from gums may only be seen in the minority of patients who still have their own teeth. Royston's curls, tightly curled body hairs caused by follicular hyperkeratosis, are said to be indicative of scurvy but unfortunately are present in many healthy old people at sites of friction from clothing, for example cuff or belt areas, and are thus a highly unreliable sign.

Diagnosis can be confirmed by the finding of a very low level of leucocyte ascorbic acid and by the rapid response to treatment with vitamin C. The vitamin C saturation test is thought to be far from reliable but is fairly easy to perform. Treatment may utilise generous doses of ascorbic acid as this is a very safe drug. Treatment should be followed up by careful dietetic advice so that subsequent relapse is avoided.

Vitamin D

Vitamin D intakes are often low in the elderly and osteomalacia is not rare. However it appears that lack of ultra-violet light exposure may be more relevant to its development than dietary vitamin D intake. Osteomalacia is considered more fully elsewhere (Chapter 21).

Calcium

Surveys have produced little to suggest that calcium is deficient in diets of the elderly and earlier theories that osteoporosis in the aged might be due to dietary calcium lack have not been supported by more recent work.

Potassium

Potassium deficiency seems to be relatively common in the elderly but in the main to be due to such causes of excessive loss as diuretic therapy, diarrhoea or renal disease. However, poor dietary intakes are a contributory factor, the elderly having generally rather poor intakes and a tendency to select potassium poor diets even when in hospital.

Dietary Fibre

Vegetable fibre is important in providing faecal bulk on which normal intestinal motility depends. The elderly commonly eat diets that supply very little roughage by reasons of habit, preference and poorer masticatory efficiency. Constipation is a very common consequence and generally responds excellently to the addition of bran to their diet.

OBESITY

Obesity is, without doubt, the commonest form of malnutrition in the elderly. It is particularly common in the elderly female where it seems not to be associated with excessive mortality although it gives rise to a great deal of morbidity such as osteoarthritis of the knees, diabetes, intertrigo and respiratory complications. In elderly men, obesity is still responsible for increased mortality and consequently has a lower prevalence.

Although obesity is clearly due to an excessive calorie intake in the past, present calorie intake may not be particularly high, indeed if obesity has resulted in disability and reduced activity, intake may be below average. In such circumstances, weight reduction is particularly difficult as a substantial cut needs to be made in a calorie intake which is already fairly low. Many obese elderly subjects will thus require their intakes to be cut to substantially less than 1000 calories if they are to lose weight at a satisfactory rate. Fortunately the elderly who need most to lose weight have already developed troublesome symptoms such as painful knees which are restricting their mobility and threatening their independence so that they are often well motivated in contrast to younger obese subjects who need to be persuaded to accept present self-denial merely to forestall potential future ills.

Further Reading

Exton-Smith, A N & Caird, F I (Eds) (1980) Metabolic and nutritional disorders in the elderly, John Wright & Sons, Bristol.

13

Mental Disturbance in Old Age

NORMAL AGEING CHANGES

Abnormal mental changes in the elderly occur against the background of insidious mental changes which can be considered to be normal. For example, reaction time becomes longer with increasing age and this seems to relate to lengthening of central reaction time and to be particularly marked where there are several alternative reactions possible.

There are also considerable changes in learning and memory, it being common knowledge that recent memory is far less efficient in old age whereas long-term memory still functions well. Learning in the young is characterised by its speed and the capacity for perfect recall. In contrast, learning in the elderly tends to be slower and to involve more reliance on the integration of new material into the framework of past learning. Older subjects have particular difficulty in learning new methods where this involves discarding or substantially altering well established methods already learned. The elderly are more likely to become anxious or to be over-cautious when faced with unfamiliar learning tasks but this is less so when learning skills have been kept sharp by regular practice.

Intelligence

There are undoubtedly changes in intelligence with age but these are not a straightforward decline. Cross-sectional studies have falsely emphasised decline of intelligence at higher ages. Longitudinal studies, in contrast, indicate that there is no progressive fall of intelligence with age provided that the individual remains in good health. However intelligence ratings may fall rapidly when ill health supervenes and a fall in mental performance may be the earliest sign of this impending deterioration in physical health.

Although overall intelligence does appear to be well preserved into advanced old age, given good physical health, there are demonstrable changes in different aspects of intellectual function. Abstract types of activity, such as solving of problems and puzzles or arithmetic, tend to reach a peak in early adult life and then slowly decline in subsequent age groups. In contrast, intelligence functions related to experience, information or vocabulary tend to continue to improve into old age. In other words, there is a tendency with increasing age to replace "fluid" by "crystallised" mental abilities so that there is a qualitative rather than a quantitative change in intelligence.

Personality

It is said that the old person grows to be more like himself, that is personality traits often become exaggerated in old age. There is a general tendency towards greater rigidity, caution, possessiveness and suspiciousness. Anxiety also appears to be more common but this may largely reflect the adversities of old age. The elderly tend to become less extraverted, to exhibit disengagement, to narrow their field of interest and to become emotionally more cool and withdrawn. They come to rely increasingly on habit and routine and because of this reliance to be more apprehensive when threatened with change.

PATHOLOGICAL MENTAL CHANGES IN THE ELDERLY

Mental impairment is a common and important problem in the aged. Community surveys have shown a high prevalence of psychiatric disability, much of it unknown to the general practitioners, while long-stay care of the elderly in hospitals and in old people's homes very largely relates to their mental disabilities. A particularly important aspect of geriatric psychiatry is the close interdependence of physical and mental disease.

The major mental disorders of the elderly can be classified under the following four headings:
1. confusional states
2. organic psychoses
3. affective disorders
4. senile paraphrenia.

Confusional States

It is in the confusional states that the close interrelationship between physical and mental illness in the elderly is most clearly seen, the confusional state often replacing fever or other physical symptoms and signs as the major presenting feature of physical illness in an elderly person.

Typically a confusional state occurs as mental disturbance of more or less sudden onset in a patient who is obviously ill, but in other instances the mental picture may be predominant and physical illness then needs to be carefully sought for if it is not to be overlooked. This is very important for, with effective treatment of the underlying physical cause, confusional states have excellent prospects for a full mental recovery.

The fully developed psychiatric picture of the confusional state is that of delirium with clouding of consciousness, gross short term memory disturbance, visual hallucinations, mood changes and behavioural disturbance. However, in the elderly incomplete clinical pictures are commonly encountered, few patients exhibiting clouding of consciousness and very few experiencing hallucinations. So it is usually not possible to distinguish confusional states from other causes of confusion on the basis of the quality of symptoms—their duration is a far better guide, recent onset of confusion pointing strongly to the diagnosis. An enormous variety of physical illnesses may present as a confusional state but particularly potent causes are infections, especially pneumonia or urinary tract infection, heart failure and carcinomatosis (Hodkinson, 1973). Acute stroke may also present as a confusional state and may give rise to diagnostic difficulty where neurological signs are few or are absent. Drug intoxications are another important group of causes. The anti-parkinsonian drugs are particularly likely to produce confusional states, especially the older atropine-like drugs such as benzhexol (artane) and orphenadrine (disipal) but the newer preparations are not blameless and amantadine may give particularly florid hallucinations. Barbiturate night sedatives have a deservedly bad reputation in elderly patients and tranquillisers too may produce confusional states when used injudiciously. The tricyclic antidepressants such as imipramine and amytriptyline are also potent causes of confusional states.

Metabolic causes of confusional states include diabetic precoma and hypoglycaemic episodes, uraemia, hepatic failure and myxoedema. Anaemia seldom results in confusional states except when very severe but B_{12} deficiency may be responsible irrespective of accompanying anaemia.

Although confusional states can occur in old people who are mentally normal, it seems that pre-existing dementia or the presence of parkinsonism serve to predispose the individual to the development of confusional states (Hodkinson, 1973).

Treatment of Confusional States. The essential of treatment is the proper recognition and prompt treatment of the underlying physical illness. Effective management of these ill, disturbed patients calls for a particularly high standard of nursing care. Where disturbed behaviour is severe, sedation may be unavoidable but as a general policy should be minimised or avoided completely. Sympathetic nursing in quiet surroundings with positive efforts to assist the patient's reorientation, particularly during periods of relatively good lucidity, help to achieve this aim. Keeping the room well lit may be helpful where there is severe nocturnal restlessness. As a general principle, unnecessary changes of staff or surroundings should be avoided so as to aid reorientation.

Organic Psychoses

Persistent confusion resulting from diffuse structural brain damage most commonly results from either senile dementia, which is a diffuse neuronal degeneration, or from damage consequent upon vascular disease, usually termed arteriosclerotic dementia though perhaps better described by the alternative term multi-infarct dementia which more satisfactorily reflects the underlying pathology. In physically fit demented elderly patients such as are admitted to mental hospitals, post mortem studies show that most can be clearly allocated to diagnostic categories of senile or arteriosclerotic or to a combination of the two. However it is unwise to assume that the same is necessarily true for ill, chronically confused patients such as those more commonly admitted to geriatric care. Some of these apparently demented subjects may rather be examples of persistent confusional states in association with chronic physical disease. Post (1978) clearly points to the need for further evaluation of the possible role of chronic confusional states in the causation of persistent confusion in ill old people.

The term dementia implies a progressive and generally irreversible global deterioration of mental function. Provided that it is recognised that in the occasional case at least, for example dementia in myxoedema or B_{12} deficiency, the condition may be reversible, the term remains a useful one. It seems an unnecessary complication to replace it with such cumbersome alternatives as chronic organic brain syndrome purely because of this semantic difficulty. However, it is very important that the label of dementia, carrying such negative associations, is not applied to patients indiscriminately. It is essential that potentially treatable conditions such as acute or chronic confusional states or depression should be recognised and that dementia is not used as a "dustbin" diagnosis for any elderly confused patient.

Senile Dementia. This is a major cause of dementia in the older age-groups, particularly in aged women. The pathological changes in the brain are indistinguishable from those of Alzheimer's disease, a genetically determined pre-senile dementia, and consist of neurofibrillary tangles and "senile plaques". It has been suggested that senile dementia too has a similar genetic basis (see review by Dayan, 1978). Plaques and tangles cannot be regarded as specific to senile dementia and Alzheimer's disease however for they also occur in Down's syndrome and in the brains of intellectually well preserved old people. However, in the latter case they are few in number whereas in senile dementia they are frequent and their number can be related to the severity of the dementia.

Recent work (see review by Bowen & Davison, 1978) has shown that the structural changes in senile dementia are accompanied by more extensive biochemical alterations, in particular a deficiency of the enzyme choline acetyl transferase. This suggests that metabolic changes in the cholinergic neurones of the brain may precede morphological changes and be a central phenomenon in the development of senile dementia. These findings open up exciting therapeutic possibilities though at the present time no effective therapy for senile dementia has been found.

The clinical picture of senile dementia is typically that of a very prolonged, steadily progressive mental decline. Memory, especially for recent events, is conspicuously impaired. There is loss of ability to concentrate and motivation deteriorates. Confabulation may be used to cover memory gaps or a good social facade may be preserved with quite skilled avoidance of answers which reveal the memory loss. The use of simple tests of orientation and memory (Hodkinson, 1972) often reveals gross impairment in subjects who pass for normal in superficial social exchanges. As dementia progresses there is increasing disorientation and disruption of thought processes. Obvious confusion and illogical thought becomes apparent. Restlessness, wandering, blunting of emotions, deterioration of personal habits and standards or apathy may be seen. Disinhibition may result in aggressive, antisocial or inappropriate sexual behaviour. The late stages of dementia are often accompanied by urinary incontinence and finally double incontinence which greatly add to the problems of care.

Some individuals may react to their developing dementia by depressive or anxiety reactions and such changes are most likely to occur in the earlier stages of the dementing process, before insight is severely impaired. Although patients with senile dementia are typically in good physical health at the outset, they none the less have a reduced life expectancy. Once dementia has become severe, life-span is usually very much shortened and physical frailty often occurs whilst respiratory infection not infrequently provides the *coup de grace*.

Arteriosclerotic Dementia. Arteriosclerotic dementia or multi-infarct dementia results from loss of brain substance from multiple infarcts secondary to thrombosis, haemorrhage or embolisation of the cerebral vessels. There is some evidence that it is the total volume of infarcted brain which determines the degree of dementia and that there is a critical volume of loss, estimated at about 50 ml, beyond which dementia is likely to result.

The clinical picture of arteriosclerotic dementia tends to differ from that of senile dementia in that progress may be by stepwise rather than steady deterioration. Furthermore there may be more day to day variation in mental symptoms, so-called arteriosclerotic variability. Arteriosclerotic dementia affects males more than females and may be associated with hypertension. The general course and manifestations of arteriosclerotic dementia otherwise closely resemble those of senile dementia, indeed are often indistinguishable. Termination may be due to a major cerebro-vascular accident or other arteriosclerotic catastrophe but more often is due to intercurrent illness of an unrelated kind. Physical examination in arteriosclerotic dementia will typically reveal bilateral pyramidal signs although these are not invariable.

Dementia in association with signs of parkinsonism is fairly commonly seen in the elderly and this is often classified as arteriosclerotic dementia. However there is no good evidence that parkinsonism in old age is in fact of arteriosclerotic origin and it is perhaps preferable to regard parkinsonism-dementia as a separate entity which typically has a very poor prognosis.

Other causes of dementia in the elderly which are occasionally encountered include dementia in association with carcinoma, neurosyphilis, "normal pressure hydrocephalus" and cerebral tumour.

Management of Dementia. There is as yet no effective treatment for the common dementias of the elderly although this has not prevented a succession of transient therapeutic enthusiasms for vitamins, procaine, RNA, folic acid, B_{12} and the current vogue for cerebral vasodilators. Drug therapy is only of symptomatic value. Restlessness can be helped by the judicious use of tranquillisers and promazine (sparine) or thioridazine (melleril) are popular choices. Depressive reactions may be helped by tricyclic anti-depressants such as amitriptyline or nortriptyline. Nocturnal restlessness may be helped by mild hypnotics such as meprobamate (equanil). Demented patients are unreliable pill takers and some may refuse all oral medication. In such instances, sedation by periodic injections of an injectable depot phenothiazine, fluphenazine (modecate), can be of value but dosage needs to be cautious initially if over-sedation and parkinsonian side effects are to be avoided.

All psychotropic drugs used in dementia are double edged weapons for if used too freely they may readily result in super-added confusional states making mental disturbance worse or may result in dangerous over-sedation and its sequelae of dehydration, pressure sores or hypostatic pneumonia.

Far more important than drug therapy is the general management of the demented elderly person. Most elderly dements are cared for in their own homes, although in some instances this may place very great stress on the caring relatives. Stress seems to occur most readily where the relationships between the old person and the caring relatives were poor before the onset of dementia; where relationships were good families may tolerate very heavy burdens uncomplainingly. The family can often be supported in a variety of ways. The general practitioner can give real help by sympathetic discussion, a judicious sedation policy and by organising the provision of appropriate social services such as district nursing for bathing, help and advice regarding nursing care and provision of incontinence pads or pants. Home Help, meals on wheels, domiciliary chiropody, incontinent laundry service or attendance at a local authority day centre may all be of help. Holiday admissions to hospital or to a local authority home may give valuable relief but the potential benefit may have to be balanced against the risk of increased disturbance which may occur when a demented elderly person is moved from his familiar surroundings.

When a dementing old person remains physically active and continent and has no gross behaviour disturbance but becomes incapable of maintaining an independent existence even with the support of social services, admission to a welfare home on a permanent basis may become the best option. Unfortunately many elderly people in this sort of situation have poor insight into their mental disabilities and may refuse to accept this. A small minority of demented subjects, particularly those with behaviour disturbance or incontinence, come to require such a degree of care that hospital admission becomes essential. Where they remain physically fit and active but have behaviour disturbance they are likely to be admitted to the psychogeriatric wards of the local mental hospital whilst those with physical illness or disability are more likely to be admitted to the geriatric service. Their management in the hospital setting calls for (but unfortunately does not always receive) good physical facilities and a high standard of nursing care. As with the care of patients with confusional states, there need to be deliberate efforts to help the patient to gain orientation. Such simple measures as colour schemes to help the patient identify where he is in the ward, use of the patient's own name rather than "gran" or some such depersonalising and patronising form of address and provision of easily seen clocks and calenders as well as books, newspapers, television and radio can all play a useful part. Sedation needs to be minimised and so do restraining devices such as cot-sides because of their demoralising effect. The importance of the patient having his own clothes and some of his own personal possessions needs to be emphasised. Social interaction and activity need to be stimulated by all possible means. Nursing staff and occupational therapists should play a leading role in this but should freely involve relatives, voluntary helpers and local organisations in their efforts to provide an interesting and stimulating environment which can do so much to prevent elderly demented patients from sinking into inertia and apathy.

Affective Disorders

Depression is the most common affective disorder in old age, its incidence rising progressively with age as well as its tendency to recurrence. Depression not infrequently occurs in the setting of physical illness or disability and may be more readily overlooked in such circumstances. Bereavement is a fairly common precipitant of depression in old age but more often there is no obvious precipitating cause and the illness can be regarded as endogenous.

In many elderly patients, depression is severe and is accompanied by apathy or agitation. There are commonly ideas of guilt or delusions of physical disease such as "the bowels are blocked", or "my organs are dead inside me" or delusions of poverty, guilt or unworthiness. In others the picture may be dominated by anxiety or hypochondriasis. A distinct suicide risk is common to both classes. Talk of suicide needs to be taken very seriously, particularly when it involves actual plans as opposed to the much more common type of remark of the form "I wish the Lord would take me".

Recognition of depression in old age is often far from straightforward. Indeed the diagnosis is perhaps more often missed than any other treatable condition in the elderly. Particular difficulties are the extreme commonness of pessimistic and valetudinarian attitudes among old people and the frequent coexistence of physical disease or disability so that some degree of melancholy can be accepted as being in keeping with the patient's condition. Poor appetite and the characteristic sleep disturbance of early waking are cardinal symptoms and should be enquired into whenever the diagnosis of depression is considered a possibility. A past history of depression can be a useful pointer. Problems may arise when severe depression is accompanied by marked apathy and withdrawl, when dementia may be mistakenly diagnosed, an error that may be helped by the patient scoring poorly on mental tests of the orientation and memory type because of poor motivation and severe withrawl.

Drug induced depression needs to be kept in mind as a possibility. Reserpine is the chief offender and may result in very severe depression requiring full treatment and not just discontinuation of the offending drug.

Treatment of Depression. The results of the treatment of depression in the elderly compare favourably with those in younger age-groups so that treatment should be given even when depression occurs in the setting of serious physical disease. Very severely depressed patients and those with marked delusions or with suicide plans are probably best treated in specialised psychiatric units, but the majority of cases can be dealt with at home or in geriatric or general wards.

The most favoured treatment method is the use of tricyclic antidepressants. Imipramine and nortriptyline are the most commonly used and there is little to chose between them except that nortriptyline is somewhat more sedating. Both may give troublesome side effects, notably postural hypotension, confusional states and atropine-like effects such as drying of the mouth, blurring of vision and the precipitation of acute retention. Because of these it is usual to start with a low dose of 30mg/day for two weeks and to increase thereafter up to a maximum of around 150mg/day until a good therapeutic response has been obtained. A response is usually seen only after a minimum of two weeks of treatment and correspondingly it is important to try the treatment for at least 4-6 weeks before abandoning it as ineffective. Once a good response has been obtained, treatment needs to be maintained, although dosage may be somewhat reduced, for at least several months and perhaps preferably for up to three years.

The newer tetracyclic antidepressants are claimed to have fewer side effects than the tricyclics but have yet to be clearly shown to be superior to them. The monoamine-oxidase inhibitor drugs are now little used because of their serious toxic effects and there is an impression that they are in any case less effective. A more useful alternative, particularly where the response delay of tricyclic therapy is undesirable because of the severity of the depression or suicide risk, is electro-convulsive therapy (E.C.T.). This is also to be considered when tricyclics have proved ineffective or poorly tolerated. Modern modified E.C.T., that is given under the cover of brief intravenous anaesthesia and muscle relaxants, can be considered even in frail or ill old people. It should be strongly considered where there is a past history of a good response to E.C.T. during a previous episode of depressive illness.

Where agitiation is prominent in a depressed patient, tranquillisers may need to be given for a time in addition to antidepressive therapy. Promazine or thioridazine are suitable choices. Night sedation may also be necessary but, in prescribing this for patients at home, the potential suicide risk needs to be kept well in mind.

Mania. Mania is comparatively rare in the elderly. Treatment is with tranquillisers or with lithium but is probably best kept in specialist psychiatric hands.

Senile Paraphrenia

The senile paraphrenics are a small group of patients, mainly women, who have well preserved if eccentric personalities and who often maintain their independence surprisingly well. They have well systematised delusions of a persecutory nature which can be very bizarre. The patient, who is often socially isolated or deaf, has little insight if any and tends to be well known to the local police and a thorn in the side of her neighbours! The condition is an intractable one although the delusions may be damped down by treatment with phenothiazines and where these are not reliably taken orally, regular injections of fluphenazine may be of value.

Alcoholism

Alcoholism is a relatively common problem in both sexes in old age though its prevalence appears to vary widely between different communities. Some elderly patients have been life-long alcoholics but a substantial number acquire the problem in old age. Alcoholism may occur in response to loneliness, bereavement, occult depressive illness or other emotional, social or medical stresses. Alcoholism should be remembered as a possible cause of incontinence, falls, confusional states and accidents as well as of other more obvious clinical manifestations such as cirrhosis or peripheral neuropathy.

Further Reading

Pitt, B (1974) Psychogeriatrics: an introduction to the clinical psychiatry of old age, Churchill Livingstone, Edinburgh.

14

Chest Disease

In old age one may encounter practically all chest disorders to be found in middle life so that this chapter cannot hope to be in any way comprehensive. It will instead deal with the chest conditions which are particularly common or important and those where the clinical picture or natural history show major differences.

Respiratory disease is very common in the elderly and this high incidence and prevalence is set against a background of age changes in the respiratory system. Pathologically, the elderly lung is lighter and shows loss of the elastic fibres whose function is to maintain the patency of small airways. In consequence there is a progressive fall of vital capacity and of forced expiratory volume (FEV_1) with age whilst residual volume increases. There is also deterioration in lung compliance, presumably due to such changes as calcification of the costal cartilages and arthritis of costo-vertebral joints leading to stiffening of the rib cage. Thoracic deformities become more common, particularly kyphosis, often consequent upon vertebral osteoporotic collapse. Respiratory function may also be affected by non-respiratory disease, for example impaired respiratory movement due to stroke or parkinsonism. Coughing tends to be less efficient and predisposes to respiratory infection and it is speculated that less effective ciliary action in old age may also contribute to this increased vulnerability.

RESPIRATORY INFECTION

The elderly seem to be particularly prone to the development of respiratory infections which are a very important cause of both morbidity and mortality in the age group. Indeed something like half of post-mortem examinations in geriatric patients show bronchopneumonic changes of some degree.

There are some important differences in the clinical features in comparison to those in middle life. Most striking perhaps is the very considerable incidence of associated confusional states with all forms of respiratory infection but especially where there is pneumonic consolidation. Another important difference is that clinical pictures are generally far less obvious and dramatic. Fever and leucocytosis are quite often absent whilst cough may be unobtrusive and pleurisy is less often encountered. The presentation is often as a very non-specific deterioration where slight dyspnoea and a raised pulse rate may be important but readily overlooked pointers to the diagnosis of chest infection. Chest infection may quite often precipitate heart failure and combined pictures of left ventricular failure and respiratory infection may be difficult to distinguish from either condition alone and it may be impossible to say which was primary and which secondary.

The difficulties of diagnosis of chest infection are compounded by those of adequately examining the chest in ill old people. Some degree of emphysema, old fibrosis or pleural thickening and chest deformity can make assessment and interpretation of signs far more difficult whilst the common occurence of basal crepitations even in well old people makes this finding particularly ambiguous.

Bronchopneumonia

Bronchopneumonic infections are particularly common and important. One form is that of terminal or "hypostatic" pneumonia which is so very frequent as the final event in debilitated old patients. Aspiration is an important mechanism in the development of bronchopneumonia and such factors as recumbency, loss of the protection of the cough reflex due to anaesthesia or over-sedation or dysphagia in such conditions as motor neurone disease, pseudobulbar palsy, stroke or severe parkinsonism or in association with obstructive lesions of the oesophagus such as cancer or stricture, are important. Vomiting or reflux are added risk factors.

Equally however, bronchopneumonia may occur suddenly in previously well and active old people, viral infection perhaps providing the trigger in some such cases.

Bronchopneumonia may pursue a rapid clinical course when left untreated so that prompt recognition and the institution of treatment without delay are essentials. Prognosis in previously well patients is good but where bronchopneumonia occurs in the setting of increasing debility, response to treatment is far less likely.

Lobar Pneumonia

Although considerably less common than bronchopneumonia, lobar pneumonia is none the less of major occurrence in the elderly. Even when extensive consolidation is present the clinical picture may still be misleadingly unobtrusive, only a proportion of cases presenting more classically with pleuritic pain, cough, rusty sputum and fever. Most often Pnuemococci are responsible but Friedlander's bacillus or Staphylococci account for some cases and produce severe illness with a marked tendency for the infection to go on to abscess formation.

Bronchitis and Emphysema

Acute bronchitis usually occurs as an exacerbation of chronic bronchitis and emphysema although it may occur independently. Severe bronchitis and emphysema, such as forms an important part of the total medical work in late middle age, particularly in men, is decidedly infrequent. The obvious explanation is that severe cases die off in late middle life and do not generally reach the geriatric age-group. However, more modest degrees of bronchitis and emphysema are common, the clinical picture being essentially similar to that in middle age. Asthma may be associated with exacerbations but cor pulmonale is unusual, perhaps because of the relative rarity of severe cases.

Even in old age, smoking remains an important adverse factor and it is still generally worthwhile to try to persuade patients to give up the habit.

Empyema

Empyema is an occasional complication of chest infections in the elderly but has special importance because of the ease with which the diagnosis may be missed and of the serious consequences of this failure. Again the problem is that of unobtrusiveness for often there may be no fever or pleuritic pain but insidious deterioration instead. Any pleural effusion in an elderly patient with chest infection or in those with heart failure who quietly lose ground should come under suspicion. Diagnostic tapping using an ordinary syringe and needle is such a quick and easy investigation that it should be freely employed so that the opportunity to treat empyema and avoid unnecessary serious deterioration or preventable death is not missed.

Treatment of Respiratory Infection

Chemotherapy of respiratory infections needs to be prompt. Soluble penicillin remains an effective treatment for many pneumonias but in very severe infections, pneumonia developing after admission to hospital and for exacerbations of chronic bronchitis, broad spectrum chemotherapy is to be preferred. Amoxycillin or cotrimoxazole are suitable choices. Therapy often has to be started in advance of bacteriological results becoming available. It is often difficult to obtain satisfactory sputum specimens in ill old people and in these circumstances blood cultures are frequently helpful.

Physiotherapy can play a useful role in treatment, assisted coughing, postural drainage and deep-breathing exercises assisting expectoration. Bronchial suction may be necessary in very ill patients.

Oxygen therapy is indicated in more severe infections particularly when anoxia leads to the development of a confusional state but may then be difficult to administer. In those with significant emphysema, the risk of increased carbon dioxide retention must be remembered and lower flow rates may be advisable.

Where heart failure complicates chest infection, energetic treatment with digitalis and diuretics should be given but can usually be discontinued once the infection has been effectively treated. Asthma in association with infection usually responds to intravenous aminophylline or the use of oral theophylline preparations such as choledyl. Troublesome cough may need suppression with linctus codeine or other opiates but the dangers of excessive respiratory depression must be avoided by careful dosage.

Hypostatic or terminal pneumonia has been called "the old man's friend" because it can so often provide a peaceful end with clouding of consciousness and finally coma in chronic debilitating illness. The doctor caring for such a deteriorating patient may thus have to make the difficult decision as to whether or not he should treat chest infection when it develops. This needs to be decided in each individual case as there can be no valid general ruling. The decision is however somewhat less agonising than might appear for experience shows that treatment appears to have only the most marginal effect, mortality remaining high. None the less it is clearly wrong to run even a smallish risk of "saving" the patient from a peaceful death perhaps to leave him to suffer greater miseries. If treatment is decided upon it should be prompt and thorough; half measures are not an acceptable substitute for a proper decision to treat or not to treat.

PULMONARY TUBERCULOSIS

Pulmonary tuberculosis is not rare in the elderly and is most likely to be overlooked in this age group, indeed all too often the diagnosis is first recognised at post-mortem. Most cases are of old fibro-caseous disease and the classical situation for the diagnosis to remain overlooked is in the old man who has chronic bronchitis as well and coughs his tubercle bacilli around the community for years with no X-ray of the chest ever being taken. Indeed his disease may only come to light when he is examined as a contact of a new case that has developed as a result.

Miliary tuberculosis is also seen occasionally and may produce an un-dramatic picture, so called "cryptic" miliary tuberculosis, the patient deteriorates slowly with general malaise and weight loss but little else and with far from obvious changes in the chest X-ray.

Treatment differs little from that in other age groups except that bed rest needs to be avoided and streptomycin should be omitted if this is possible as it so commonly results in serious ototoxicity in the elderly.

PULMONARY FIBROSIS

Pneumoconioses are rare but the occasional case of asbestosis is seen with pulmonary fibrosis accompanied by the give-away sign of patches of pleural calcification and often relates to minor exposure very many years previously. Chronic intestitial pulmonary fibrosis in association with rheumatoid arthritis is the commonest type of pulmonary fibrosis seen and typically occurs in long-standing sero-positive cases.

CANCER OF THE LUNG

Carcinoma of the bronchus ranks as one of the most common cancers of the elderly. Both the male preponderance and the association with smoking become less striking in old age. Squamous histological types of growth predominate, anaplastic ("oat" cell) types are next most frequent and only about one in twenty are adenocarcinomata.

The presentation is very varied, weight loss and cough, haemoptysis, obstructive pneumonia, dyspnoea or other pulmonary symptoms being the most common. Pleural effusion, lung abscess or superior vena caval obstruction are other important presentations. In many patients, however, the disease may only become manifest when distant metastasis has occured, cerebral metastasis being particularly associated with adenocarcinoma and bone and hepatic metastases with the squamous and anaplastic tumours. Toxic confusional states are another possible presentation. Less common but important modes of presentation are pulmonary osteopathy, neuropathies such as peripheral neuropathy, cerebellar neuropathy or dementia and metabolic syndromes due to secretion of hormone-like peptides such as hypercalcaemia due to parathormone-like activity.

Treatment is particularly unsatisfactory in the elderly. Operative mortality is much higher even in the minority who are fit enough for surgery to be undertaken. Even in younger patients operative results are very poor and appear worse than those of radiotherapy so that surgery in old age should probably be ruled out. Radiotherapy itself carries a very high morbidity and only a very small hope of "cure". It is therefore perhaps best to restrict its use to those patients who have troublesome symptoms which radiotherapy can effectively relieve and not to attempt radical treatment in other cases. The best case for radiotherapy is thus in the palliation of superior vena caval obstruction or of painful bony deposits where gratifying results may be obtained.

Apart from carcinoma of the bronchus, secondary lung cancer is frequent. Multiple lung deposits seen on chest X-ray may reveal the diagnosis of carcinomatosis in patients showing only a general mental and physical deterioration. Common primary sources for pulmonary secondary deposits are cancers of breast and of the gastro-intestinal tract and primary lung cancer itself may often show lung metastases.

15

Heart Disease

Heart disease plays a very large part in clinical geriatrics, cardiac failure accounting for about 15 per cent of admissions to geriatric departments for example. Most heart diseases, even including congenital lesions, are to be found in old age and may show little difference in their clinical expression compared to that in the young. This chapter will concentrate on the more common and important conditions, particularly where the clinical picture is modified by age.

A number of changes are commonly found in the elderly heart. Some degree of muscle atrophy, the deposition of increasing amounts of the age pigment lipofuscin and an increase in collagenous fibrous tissue can perhaps be considered as normal age changes. Perhaps more clearly pathological are such changes as mitral ring calcification, mucoid degeneration of the mitral valve ('floppy' valve), calcification of the aortic valve cusps and senile cardiac amyloidosis, all of which are to be found virtually exclusively in old age however.

ISCHAEMIC HEART DISEASE

Ischaemic heart disease is probably the most important class of heart disease in the elderly. Incidence and prevalence rise with age and the male preponderance becomes progressively less marked.

Myocardial Infarction

Acute myocardial infarction is very common in old age in males and females alike. The clinical picture is very often modified. Only a minority present typically with severe chest pain and shock. An important presentation is the insidious development of increasing dyspnoea or onset of attacks of left ventricular failure or of congestive cardiac failure. Syncopal attacks, prostration and extreme weakness or associated stroke or arterial embolism are other possible presentations. Confusional states are another quite common clinical picture, sometimes taking the form of repeated nocturnal confusion associated with episodes of nocturnal dyspnoea. Other infarcts may result in sudden death but, at the other extreme, it seems clear that many myocardial infarctions in the elderly are completely silent for there is often post-mortem or electrocardiographic evidence of old infarction in the absence of any matching clinical history.

Management of myocardial infarction should avoid the use of bed rest because of its considerable risks. A period of 7-10 days of chair rest is usually employed instead. Arrhythmias call for prompt treatment and Coronary Care Unit management is of benefit in complicated cases. There is no real indication that routine or long-term anticoagulant therapy are of any value in elderly pateints with myocardial infarction and most geriatricians only employ a course of anticoagulation where complicating deep vein thrombosis or pulmonary embolism have been diagnosed.

Myocardial infarction has quite a good prognosis in the aged when considered in relationship to the general prognosis in the age group. It is therefore realistic to adopt a reasonably optimistic attitude in management and in particular to make every effort to dissuade patients from a subsequent life of unnecessary invalidism.

Angina Pectoris

This generally good prognosis extends to that of angina pectoris which is in any event rather less often met with in the elderly than would be expected on the basis of the frequency of other manifestations of ischaemic heart disease. This may be due partly to the alteration of pain mechanisms, already seen in the comparatively common occurence of painless myocardial infarction, but also because reduced capacity for physical exertion may preclude its development. Anginal pain may be rather atypical in its character and dyspnoea rather than pain may be the major limiting factor in determining exercise tolerance. Differential diagnosis includes such possibilities as hiatus hernia and gall-stones but an occasional pitfall is costo-chondral pain (Tietze's syndrome) which may produce quite severe episodes of pain during activity but which is accompanied by exquisite pain over the offending joint. This is particularly seen in old patients who have rheumatoid arthritis.

Where angina is troublesome, trinitrin is often helpful but long-acting coronary vasodilators appear to be quite useless. As in the case of myocardial infarction it is important to encourage patients to lead as active a life as possible for cardiac neurosis is frequently a far more troublesome disease than is ischaemic heart disease itself. In this regard, a useful therapeutic device which may enable patients to maintain some useful activity which tends to provoke an anginal attack is to routinely use trinitrin just before the activity is undertaken. It can then sometimes be habitually carried out without angina.

VALVULAR DISEASE OF THE HEART

Valvular disease is quite common in old age. Rheumatic heart disease accounts for a substantial proportion, degenerative processes are important whilst congenital defects such as atrial septal defects and aortic valve abnormalities may still be encountered occasionally. Comprehensive post-mortem studies have done much to elucidate the pathology of valvular disease in old age and have shown that lesions are often multiple and that few murmurs in the old are truly "insignificant".

Mitral Valve Disease

Bedford and Caird (1960) found mitral disease in some 4 per cent of geriatric patients, incompetence being more frequent than stenosis as the predominant lesion. The mitral disease often leads to cardiac failure and the physical signs closely resemble those in the young. Surgical treatment of the more severe mitral valve lesions can still be a worthwhile proposition for patients well into the seventh decade.

Mitral ring calcification, believed to be of degenerative rather than rheumatic aetiology, is also quite common. Although minor degrees are essentially asymptomatic, more severe changes may produce mitral systolic murmurs or even functionally significant mitral incompetence (or rarely stenosis) and can also provide the basis for the development of subacute bacterial endocarditis.

Aortic Valve Disease

Calcific aortic valve disease is very common but only results in functional aortic stenosis in a minority of cases. The remaining cases with aortic ejection murmurs but no functional stenosis of significance are often distinguished by the designation aortic sclerosis. The clinical differentiation of the two may be difficult in practice however. True aortic stenosis results in marked left ventricular hypertrophy and the risk of sudden death, syncopal attacks or the development of left ventricular failure or congestive cardiac failure. Its diagnosis should thus depend on the demonstration of left ventricular hypertrophy clinically, electrocardiographically or radiologically in the presence of the characteristic aortic systolic murmur which is typically loud. The classical small and delayed pulse is often absent and pulse pressure may not be particularly small and the absence of these findings by no means excludes the diagnosis. Reversed splitting and reduced intensity of the second heart sound may provide a useful confirmatory sign. The general effect of these difficulties is that aortic stenosis tends to be under-diagnosed and too many aortic ejection murmurs accepted as being benign.

The aetiology of aortic stenosis is probably mainly degenerative although a minority of cases are probably rheumatic. Aortic incompetence on the other hand is most often rheumatic, syphilis being a rare cause these days. However a substantial minority of cases fall into a category referred to as "isolated" aortic incompetence. These cases have no associated aortic stenosis and no evidence of syphilis and the degree of incompetence is often of little clinical significance, the prognosis being good. These are probably of degenerative aetiology due to aortic ring stretching. In old age the diastolic murmur of aortic incompetence is often faint and very high pitched and best heard at the left sternal edge or even at the apex rather than at the aortic area. It can very easily be missed if not listened for carefully, preferably with the patient sitting forwards.

CARDIAC ARRHYTHMIAS

The incidence of cardiac arrhythmias rises with age and all types of arrhythmia may be encountered. Minor abnormalities such as ventricular or less often supra-ventricular extrasystoles occurring occasionally or sinus arrhythmia, exaggerated variation in rate with respiration, are quite common and probably of little practical significance.

Many arrhythmias may be seen in digitalis intoxication, for example frequent ventricular extrasystoles, coupled beats, ventricular or supra-ventricular tacycardias and incomplete heart block. Sinus bradycardia may be seen occasionally in severe myxoedema and quite often occurs in hypothermia. Sinus tachycardia may accompany infections, haemorrhage, heart failure or thyrotoxicosis.

Auricular Fibrillation

The prevalence of atrial fibrillation rises with age and can be related to the gradual increase in fibrous tissue within the conducting system. It is also associated with ischaemic heart disease, valvular lesions, particularly floppy mitral valve, and with senile cardiac amyloidosis (Hodkinson & Pomerance, 1979). It may also be due to thyrotoxicosis or may occur transiently with acute respiratory infection.

In some elderly patients with atrial fibrillation the pulse rate remains quite slow so that little functional disturbance results. Fast atrial fibrillation, in contrast, has considerable effects on cardiac efficiency and often precipitates heart failure and thus requires treatment. Digitalis is the corner-stone of therapy and should usually be continued on a permanent basis. Because of impaired renal function and reduced lean body mass, many old people are so sensitive to digitalis that maintenance can more conveniently be achieved by using "paediatric" tablets of 0.0625 mg of digoxin rather than the regular 0.25 mg tablets. It is very rarely advisable to attempt to restore sinus rhythm with quinidine or electrical cardioversion except possibly in the case of fibrillation persisting after the successful treatment of thyrotoxicosis. Occasionally when control of atrial fibrillation with digitalis cannot be achieved satisfactorily propanalol may be useful but needs to be carefully monitored because of the risk of precipitating cardiac failure or postural hypotension.

Complete Heart Block

Complete heart block, where there is complete dissociation between atrial and ventricular beats so that the pulse rate depends on idio-ventricular rhythm and is thus typically slow but regular, is an important and not uncommon finding in the elderly. The ventricular rate is typically of the order of 20-50/min and with slower rates cardiac failure often results. The other important manifestation of complete block is Stokes-Adams attacks due to periods of ventricular asystole. These occur more when complete block first develops and may be alternating with other types of rhythm and are often not a feature once complete block has become established. Stokes-Adams attacks are an important cause of falls and fits and carry the risk of death if the asystole is sufficiently prolonged.

The aetiology of complete heart block in the old is not usually myocardial infarction as in the young but, especially in the chronic examples, appears to be due to localised minor fibrotic changes of uncertain origin involving the bundle of His or both bundle branches (Davies, 1971). Thus complete heart block has a generally reasonably good prognosis and makes active treatment measures potentially very rewarding.

The treatment of choice for complete heart block is the provision of an artificial pacemaker and this procedure can be considered even for very frail elderly patients.

Bundle Branch Block

Both right and left bundle branch block are common, although left bundle branch block is the more frequent of the two. They may be associated with either ischaemia or with fibrosis of unknown cause (Davies, 1971). Clinically, right bundle branch block may be associated with cor pulmonale while left block may occur with hypertension or aortic stenosis. The prognosis of bundle branch block is really that of the underlying pathology itself and where there is no apparent associated disease is good.

BACTERIAL ENDOCARDITIS

Nearly a third of cases of subacute bacterial endocarditis are now diagnosed in patients aged over sixty. The clinical picture in elderly cases is often an obscure one so that the diagnosis is probably quite frequently overlooked and the true incidence in old age correspondingly under-estimated. This is of considerable practical importance for the disease carries a very grave prognosis if left untreated while the outlook with treatment is moderately good. The disease is often of very slow and insidious onset and may give rise only to such non-specific symptoms as malaise, weight loss, mental confusion, vague aches and pains or merely a general "failure to thrive". More specifically, anaemia, fever, purpura, clubbing or embolic phenomena such as Osler's nodes, haematuria or obvious cerebral or peripheral emboli may draw attention to the possibility of the diagnosis. Certainly the diagnosis needs to be thought of in any old person with a heart murmur who deteriorates without a clear cause or who slips into cardiac failure for no apparent reason. The slightest suspicion of bacterial endocarditis calls for a series of blood cultures, preferably 4-6 in total and these should be examined for both anaerobic and aerobic growth. Streptococcus viridans is still the principal responsible organism although the disease has altered over the years (Hayward, 1973) and other organisms are now more often found than before. Only a minority of patients have had dental procedures, catheterisation or instrumentation of the urinary tract as apparent reasons for the initial bacteraemia giving rise to the disease and the mechanism in the majority remains obscure. The underlying structural abnormalities are commonly mitral valve lesions, particularly mitral incompetence but mitral ring calcification, mitral stenosis and aortic valve disease are also important.

In the case of the usual Streptococcus viridans infection, penicillin in high dosage given for at least a month or six weeks remains the treatment of choice. Injection of large amounts of penicillin in wasted old patients may present major difficulties so that the addition of oral probenecid to give higher penicillin levels for a given dose of penicillin is a useful measure. Parenteral penicillin is to be preferred but large oral doses can be an alternative, particularly in the closing stages of treatment when the patient may find continuation of intramuscular treatment increasingly hard to tolerate. Where other organisms are responsible, similar prolonged courses of the appropriate antibiotic are indicated. A not infrequent problem is when subacute bacterial endocarditis is strongly suspected on clinical ground but blood cultures are negative. In view of the seriousness of leaving the disease untreated it is probably best to give such patients the benefit of the doubt and give a full course of penicillin therapy. In patients with clear evidence of embolic phenomena it is hazardous to await the blood culture results and it is wise to begin penicillin treatment as soon as the specimens have been taken.

The need to give prophylactic penicillin cover when old patients with susceptible valvular lesions have dental treatment or other provocative surgical procedures should not be forgotten. The antibiotic needs to be started immediately before the relevant procedure is carried out.

HEART FAILURE

Heart failure is a major component of the work of a geriatric department. In a good proportion of cases the underlying cause of cardiac failure may be reasonably obvious, for example rheumatic heart disease, aortic stenosis, recent myocardial infarction or auricular fibrillation or other arrhythmia. It may be due to the effect of non-cardiac disease such as anaemia, thyrotoxicosis, cor pulmonale, extensive Paget's disease leading to high output failure or to the salt retaining effects of drugs such as stilboestrol, carbenoxolone, prednisone or phenylbutazone. However there remains a substantial group of cases where the cause of the cardiac failure is far from clear. It is tempting to ascribe these to ischaemic heart disease or to hypertension on slender evidence. Post-mortem studies rather indicate that ischaemic heart disease without actual infarction, recent or old, does not cause cardiac failure and that hypertension is not an important factor. It appears that ischaemic heart disease, atrial fibrillation and senile cardiac amyloidosis are the main pathologies associated with cardiac failure in the elderly and that their affects are often additive (Hodkinson & Pomerance, 1979). Unrecognised pulmonary emboli are an important cause of cardiac failure and repeated small emboli may cause the steady deterioration in cardiac failure due to other underlying causes despite energetic treatment.

Cardiac Amyloidosis

Cardiac amyloidosis is a common post-mortem finding in the oldest age-groups, its incidence rising to around 50 per cent in those over ninety. It is found as a fine network of deposits around myocardial muscle cells but also as small nodules in the atrial endocardium. There is usually no associated disease to which the amyloidosis could be attributed so that these cases of "senile" amyloidosis are a variety of primary amyloidosis. There is now good evidence that quite modest degrees of senile amyloidosis are associated with heart failure so that this may be quite an important occult cause of failure in the higher age-groups particularly.

THE CLINICAL PICTURE OF HEART FAILURE

The clinical features of congestive heart failure and of left ventricular failure are in general little different from those in earlier age-groups. However one special feature is that heart failure may quite commonly result in confusional states. Paroxysmal nocturnal dyspnoea may thus produce multiple episodes of nocturnal confusion. Another feature is that the elderly may often greatly delay the seeking of medical help. It is thus not rare to see very advanced cases of congestive heart failure with astounding degrees of oedema and with effusions and ascites. Another characteristic feature that is common in the old but rarely seen in the young is the development of translucent blisters on the legs. These particularly occur when, because of orthopnoea, the patient sleeps in his chair at night so that the hydrostatic pressure in his oedematous legs is never relieved. Superficial blisters filled with oedema fluid result and are often multiple and usually oval and sometimes of considerable size. They resemble the superficial blisters produced by scalding and perhaps for this reason are often falsely ascribed to the effects of sitting with the legs too near the fire by the patient or his doctor. This is clearly not so for the lesions are met only in those with severe leg oedema and often involve areas such as the dorsum of the foot which are not at risk to toasting by radiant heat from the fire. They clearly represent blistering due to excessive hydrostatic pressure in the tissues. They commonly burst spontaneously and then discharge considerable amounts of oedema fluid which can perhaps have beneficial effects, acting like a spontaneous form of acupuncture.

TREATMENT OF HEART FAILURE

The overall results of the treatment of heart failure in the elderly are generally good whilst the principles of treatment are closely similar to those in younger patients. However, the use of rest needs to be modified, chair rest taking the place of full bed rest wherever possible. Potent diuretics such as frusemide are commonly used for initial treatment but because of their rapid action may precipitate retention of urine in old men with prostatic hypertrophy. In such cases the slow acting diuretic chlorthalidone may be useful but sometimes where this is insufficient to overcome the difficulty, catheterisation during the initial phase of major diuresis may be necessary. Potassium supplements are mandatory because of the particular vulnerability of the elderly to the development of potassium depletion. Digitalis is an important aspect of treatment despite its considerable hazards. Certainly it must be used when atrial fibrillation is involved but it is not essential in milder cases of cardiac failure in sinus rhythm where there is a reasonable case for using diuretics alone.

Resistant heart failure may call for very high doses of diuretics or the adding of spironolactone to the regime may sometimes be helpful. Sometimes when such measures are unavailing there is still a case for mechanical removal of oedema fluid. Southey's tubes are unnecessary for this purpose, simple acupuncture by multiple needle pricks to the dorsum of the foot after a preparatory period of dependency of the legs gives very adequate drainage, one or two gallons draining in just a few days during which it is probably wise to maintain antibiotic cover. After this there may well be a striking improvement in response to diuretics. Energetic treatment of refractory cases may result in severe hyponatraemia and it is then necessary to restrict water intake to a maximum of a litre per day until the sodium has risen. It is also important to avoid overtreatment that leads to severe dehydration and if this occurs it may be necessary to stop diuretics for a time to allow recovery.

Once heart failure has been effectively controlled maintenance treatment will be necessary where the basic cause is irreversible, for example valvular disease, but will not be where there is a fully reversible cause such as thyrotoxicosis or anaemia. Causes such as acute myocardial infarction lead to a less predictable situation. The general aim should clearly be to cut maintenance treatment to a minimum or to completely stop treatment if at all possible. This requires careful supervision and good judgement and it needs to be remembered that a common reason for relapse is the failure of the patient to take his prescribed treatment.

Left ventricular failure as opposed to congestive heart failure may call for some modifications of therapy. It may be helpful initially to tap large pleural effusions and where nocturnal dyspnoea occurs it can be useful to give frusemide during the afternoon rather than in the morning. Nepenthe, 1 ml, as a hypnotic and aminophyllin suppositories at bed-time may also help to prevent the nocturnal attacks. Sudden severe attacks of left ventricular failure call for the use of intravenous frusemide and heroin, 10 mg, adds greatly to the effectiveness of treatment and may be given half subcutaneously and the remainder intravenously. Intravenous aminophyllin, 0.5 g, may also give a little additional help but where these treatments still fail to control the attack, the effects of either venous cuffing of the legs or venesection can be life saving.

MANAGEMENT OF CARDIAC ARREST

The temptation to use the "crash call" team to attempt to resuscitate elderly patients in whom cardiac arrest occurs needs to receive careful consideration. There is absolutely no merit in attempting to resuscitate patients who had been pursuing a steadily downhill course before the arrest or who were known to be likely to die soon. There should, in other words, be no attempt to postpone an inevitable death nor to try to prolong a life which entails further suffering without hopes of recovery. On the other hand, resuscitation should not be witheld purely because a patient is elderly provided that they had a good prognosis prior to the arrest and thus have hope of full recovery if the attempt is successful. The attempt must be a very prompt one if the therapeutic tragedy of a virtually decerebrate survivor is to be avoided and even with prompt intervention the success rate is low in the elderly. A further consideration is that some old patients and their families have strong views against resuscitation, fear of which may on occasions lead to refusal of the offer of admission to hospital when this is medically indicated. In practice, resuscitation attempts in geriatric wards tend to be very few and far between.

16

Blood Pressure, Arterial Disease and Thromboembolism

ARTERIAL BLOOD PRESSURE

Hypotension

Disturbances of autonomic function are common in old age (Exton-Smith, 1978) and postural hypotension is a common consequence. Postural hypotension is often worse in the morning and occurs when the patient stands up from the sitting or especially from the lying position. It may not develop immediately but take up to a minute or so and its onset is favoured by exertion such as walking. The initial blood pressure may be raised or normal but falls to levels where cerebral perfusion is adversely affected and giddiness, vertigo, faintness and even transient syncope result and the patient exhibits pallor and a thin pulse that may become virtually undetectable. In fact many elderly patients exhibit some fall of blood pressure on standing even though this may not give rise to symptoms whilst symptomatic cases usually have falls of diastolic pressure of 20mm Hg or more.

Postural hypotension is favoured by prolonged recumbency, yet another reason for minimising bed rest in the treatment of the elderly. In many patients, defective baroreceptor reflexes are demonstrable and these neurological abnormalities are particularly found where there is cerebrovascular disease such as stroke or Parkinsonism. In addition many other factors may operate, important among these are conditions leading to impairment of cardiac output such as salt depletion, aortic stenosis, recent myocardial infarction, pulmonary embolism or gastrointestinal haemorrhage. Severe infection or anaemia are further possibilities and drugs are often implicated. Examples of drugs giving rise to postural hypotension are anti-hypertensive agents, sedatives, tranquillisers, potent diuretics and anti-cholinergic drugs such as tricyclic antidepressants, anti-parkinsonian drugs and antihistamines.

Management consists of treating associated disease conditions or the withdrawal of provocative drugs plus general measures. Patients should avoid further unnecessary recumbency for this often results in further impairment. It appears that reflex vasomotor control is amenable to some degree of re-education so that patients should be encouraged to alter posture frequently. So as not to precipitate symptoms unduly, they should be advised to do this slowly, first sitting on the edge of the bed for a short while and then standing up in a unhurried manner. Full length elastic stockings, put on before rising from bed and worn all day, may give some assistance by reducing the tendency for blood to pool in the legs. Where salt depletion is a factor, salt supplements should be given or fludrocortisone may be used.

Hypertension

Blood pressure tends to rise with age although the rate of increase seems to fall off beyond sixty-five and may even be reversed in the oldest age-groups. This may be because severe hypertension has been largely eliminated in the earlier age-groups because of its lethal effects.

It is not possible to give a firm ruling as to what should be accepted as a "normal" blood pressure in old age. Certainly the standards can be less strict than in younger patients and purely systolic hypertension is to be disregarded in practical terms although it is probably an indication of decreased vascular elasticity. A diastolic level of 110 mm Hg or more can reasonably be taken as hypertensive if this is sustained under conditions which do not produce stress or anxiety. This rider is an important one for many old patients appear to have particularly labile blood pressure. They may have high blood pressure readings when first examined or at casual repeat readings and be mistakenly diagnosed as hypertensive while regular daily charting of the blood pressure shows that the high early readings settle down to perfectly acceptable values after a few days. It is therefore essential that such an assessment should be made before hypertension is diagnosed in any old person and is absolutely mandatory where treatment is contemplated. If these precautions are always observed, the frequency of hypertension is found to be far less than is commonly thought.

Hypertension in the elderly is almost always "essential", for very few cases indeed are due to such causes as Cushing's syndrome, phaeochromocytoma or renal lesions and malignant hypertension is extremely rare.

Consequences of Hypertension. Hypertension seems to have less serious effects in the old in comparison with the young. Elderly women in particular seem to be capable of withstanding moderate hypertension for long periods with apparent impunity. The effects seen are mainly those attributable to secondary arterial disease, particularly strokes and myocardial infarction but renal damage is not a prominent feature. Some patients with more severe levels of hypertension may develop a rather rapidly progressive arteriosclerotic dementia or pseudobulbar palsy. Heart failure, particularly left ventricular failure, is another consequence but is not particularly common.

Treatment of Hypertension. Most geriatricians take the view that treatment of hypertension in old age should only be undertaken for very clear reasons. The common experience is that one more often stops such treatment started by others because of its unfortunate effects than one starts treatment in new cases.

The case for treating asymptomatic hypertension of moderate degree, particularly in the elderly female, is a very flimsy one and most geriatricians would withhold therapy. This similarly applies where such symptoms as giddiness or headache have led to the discovery of hypertension for these symptoms are most unlikely to be due to it. There is no evidence to indicate that reduction of blood pressure by treatment protects against further stroke in hypertensive patients who have already sustained a cerebrovascular accident nor that future myocardial infarction can be avoided where there is established ischaemic heart disease. Arteriosclerotic dementia, pseudobulbar palsy or renal failure are generally taken to be positive contraindications to treatment.

The clearest indications to treatment are thus in the very occasional case of malignant hypertension, where hypertension has given rise to heart failure or has given rise to signs of incipient decompensation such as gallop rhythm in association with evidence of left ventricular hypertrophy, and finally where there is hypertension of severe degree even though this may be asymptomatic. The evidence for and against treatment of less severe hypertension has recently been reviewed (Moore-Smith, 1980). Treatment usually starts with a thiazide diuretic with subsequent addition of methyl-dopa or a beta-blocker if necessary. Treatment should aim at cautious reduction of blood pressure, therapy being built up gradually in a step-wise manner. Reserpine should be avoided because of its capacity to give rise to depression whilst the powerful ganglion blocking drugs are unsuitable for use in the elderly because of the risks of postural hypotension.

Arteriosclerosis

Atherosclerosis is the major form of arteriosclerosis both in terms of prevalence and its serious consequences in old age. It underlies much of the mortality and morbidity of old age, particularly such major entities as ischaemic heart disease, stroke, arteriosclerotic dementia and peripheral vascular disease. The pathology and aetiology form an enormous and confused topic which cannot appropriately be dealt with here; the interested reader is referred to the up to date review of the subject from the geriatric standpoint by Walton (1978).

Atherosclerosis is a patchy disorder whose earliest lesions affect the intima of arteries, leading to the development of atheromatous plaques which cause narrowing of the arterial lumen and favour the occurrence of thrombosis which may thus result in total occlusion of the vessel. Hypertension, diabetes and heredity appear to be factors relevant to the development of atheroma but, although showing a strong association with age, it seems not to be a true ageing change.

Monckeberg medial sclerosis is another form of arteriosclerosis which is also strongly associated with age but has little in the way of serious consequences. Here the disease affects the media which degenerates and becomes calcified,

X-rays in old people often showing pipe-stem calcification of the complete main arterial tree from this cause.

A further age change covered by the term arteriosclerosis is the replacement of muscle in larger vessels by fibrous tissue and the general stretching of arterial walls which become both wider and longer, that is more tortuous. These changes, atheroma and medial sclerosis, very often coexist in the elderly patient.

Clinical Consequences of Atherosclerosis

The tendency is for atherosclerosis to be generalised even though the heaviest involvement may fall on one particular organ. Thus, for example, patients with peripheral vascular disease are more likely than average to also have ischaemic heart disease or cerebral arteriosclerosis. The important manifestations of atheroma, stroke, arteriosclerotic dementia, ischaemic heart disease and myocardial infarction have been dealt with elsewhere and will not be discussed further.

Peripheral Vascular Disease. Objective evidence of the impairment of arterial blood supply in the legs is quite common as shown by absent peripheral pulses, lowered skin temperature, impoverished skin nutrition with corresponding nail and hair changes, and dependent rubor or cyanosis. Despite this, intermittent claudication is not particularly common, a situation which parallels that obtaining in the case of angina pectoris. The explanation is likely to be the same, partly the alteration of pain mechanisms and partly the reduced capacity for exercise. Treatment of intermittent claudication may be surgical where justified by the severity of symptoms and interference with the life of a patient who is not too elderly. Reconstructive vascular surgery is the most helpful approach as lumbar sympathectomy gives generally disappointing results, although it can prove very useful in the treatment of ischaemic ulceration of the skin. Treatment with vasodilator drugs such as tolazoline tends to be extremely disappointing in either situation. Perhaps this is not surprising, for a vasodilator will dilate normal but not diseased vessels and may thus even reduce flow to the ischaemic area by a "steal" phenomenon. Giving up smoking is far more valuable than vasodilators.

Gangrene is the most important complication of peripheral vascular disease. This typically develops quite suddenly without warning or obvious provocative cause because of thrombosis or embolism of the main arterial supply at a far higher level than might be predicted from the extent of the gangrene. In other cases however local infection may be a precipitating factor, perhaps because of the increased oxygen demand created by the accompanying inflammatory response. The need for good foot hygiene and careful chiropody in patients with peripheral vascular disease is thus to be stressed.

Although small, well circumscribed areas of gangrene, for example confined to the great toe, may sometimes be managed successfully by conservative measures with eventual separation of the escar, perhaps with minor surgical assistance, the majority of cases of gangrene call for amputation without undue delay. There is a strong case for amputation through or above the knee even where gangrene is confined to the foot for too many below knee amputations fail to heal so that further amputation at a higher level becomes necessary to the disadvantage of the patient and his rehabilitation. The risks of surgery are far less than those of conservative management in all but the very frail, and early amputation gives generally excellent prospects for rehabilitation. Even double amputation at advanced ages is consistent with success although most patients need to keep to short "rocker" pylons because of the far greater difficulty of managing full length prostheses. Unfortunately, even though the short term prognosis and rehabilitation prospects after amputation for arteriosclerotic gangrene are generally good, the common association of other forms of arteriosclerotic disease carries a poor long-term prognosis and a distressingly high proportion of successfully treated cases die of other vascular catastrophes such as stroke or myocardial infarction within the following year or two. However this is an essentially unpredictable matter and other individuals may have years of reasonable life ahead of them so that treatment and rehabilitation should be pursued in all patients wholeheartedly. In diabetic subjects the long term prognosis is, perhaps surprisingly, distinctly better, possibly because the arterial disease is more peripheral and associated with less generally advanced atheroma elsewhere. This better prognosis is illustrated by the considerable preponderance of diabetics among those with double amputation whereas diabetics account for only a minority of first amputations.

Aortic Aneurism. This can be another manifestation of arteriosclerosis in old age and is not rare, only a small proportion of aneurisms being syphilitic nowadays. Thoracic aneurisms are often asymptomatic but if very large may give rise to a variety of pressure symptoms. Abdominal aortic aneurisms are far from rare. They carry a risk of rupture which appears to have been exaggerated in the surgical literature. Symptomless abdominal aneurisms, even if large, are probably best left alone. However, increasing size, tenderness and pain are probably quite grave prognostic signs and may make operation with prosthetic replacement of the affected part of the aorta the better choice despite its considerable mortality.

Dissecting Aneurism of the Aorta. Dissecting aneurism carries a very high immediate mortality, making a significant contribution to cases of sudden unexpected death in the elderly. Higher age, hypertension and arteriosclerosis are all factors associated with it.

The basic pathology is that bleeding into the degenerate medial coat of the aorta takes place through a spontaneous intimal tear which may be associated with an atheromatous plaque. The ensuing dissection of the aorta may also involve its branches so that a variety of ischaemic phenomena such as stroke, myocardial infarction, paraparesis or loss of peripheral pulses may occur in addition to the severe chest pain and shock due to the aortic dissection itself. Fatal cases often have massive haemorrhage into the pleura or pericardium whilst those who survive tend to do so by virtue of the development of re-entrant tears further along the aorta so that adequate flow can continue through the resultant new passage along the media. Surgical treatment is rarely a practical proposition in the elderly. The diagnosis should be considered when severe chest pain and shock suddenly develop and a characteristic widening of the aortic shadow on chest X-ray may be a useful diagnostic pointer.

THROMBOEMBOLIC DISEASE

Thromboembolism is an important disease process in old age. It may affect either the greater or lesser circulations but is far more common in the latter which will be considered first.

Venous Thrombosis and Pulmonary Embolism

Pulmonary embolism is a condition whose importance is difficult to over-emphasise in old age and which is seriously under-diagnosed in clinical practice. Postmortem studies show that recent pulmonary emboli are present in about a third of routine geriatric autopsies but that only a fraction of these were correctly diagnosed or even suspected before death.

Venous thromboses are the source of the vast majority of pulmonary emboli. Most often responsible are deep venous thromboses of the leg, though pelvic veins and veins of the prostatic bed are quite important too. Factors inducing venous stasis are thus of importance and these include immobility from bed rest, fracture, joint disease or paralysis. Venous damage from chronic venous insufficiency, fracture of the femur or surgery are important factors while metabolic disturbances such as dehydration, toxaemia or carcinomatosis may also favour thrombosis. Fracture of the femur, stoke, myocardial infarction, congestive cardiac failure and carcinomatosis are perhaps the most common clinical associations therefore.

Recognition of Venous Thrombosis. Only a small proportion of leg vein thromboses are clinically apparent, giving rise to pain, tenderness, locally raised skin temperature or a positive Homan's sign. Many thromboses are clinically undetectable yet pose the threat of pulmonary embolism. These can only be detected by use of isotope-labelled fibrinogen techniques or by venography. It is these methods that have uncovered the strikingly high incidences of venous thrombosis in ill old people and after surgery. The commonly used technique of leg scanning after radiofibrinogen administration fails to detect thrombosis above the inguinal ligament but this defect can be overcome by combined monitoring of plasma decay of I_{125} activity, fast disappearance rates indicating thrombosis (Denham *et al.*, 1973).

Recognition of Pulmonary Embolism. The recognition of pulmonary embolism is also difficult. Only a minority produce a "textbook" clinical picture of sudden collapse with chest pain, dyspnoea, cyanosis and often rapid death in the case of large emboli or pleuritic chest pain accompanied by dyspnoea and sometimes haemoptysis in the case of smaller ones. Far more often, presentation is more indefinite. Dyspnoea and tachycardia without obvious cause, worsening of heart failure, particularly when pleural effusions appear, or signs of pulmonary consolidation which do not respond to antibiotic therapy should all suggest the diagnosis. Sudden deterioration in stroke patients although often put down to the occurence of a further cerebro-vascular episode, is most usually due to pulmonary embolism. The occurrence of repeated small emboli may produce a type of cor pulmonale and lead to heart failure but more often merely results in a totally non-specific and gradual decline. Pulmonary embolism thus calls for consideration as a possible diagnosis in any elderly patient who deteriorates for no clear reason but more particularly when dyspnoea or tachycardia are present. Chest X-ray may aid diagnosis by showing characteristic wedge shaped opacities or the presence of pleural effusion. Later, typical horizontal linear opacities may appear which are strong evidence that emboli have occured. Lung scans can also be helpful, showing areas of reduced perfusion but are not always a practicable investigation in ill old people.

Treatment of Venous Thrombosis and Pulmonary Embolism. Because of the associated morbidity and mortality, venous thrombosis and pulmonary embolism are the most important indications for anticoagulant therapy in old age. Similar regimes to those in younger age groups can be employed such as heparin for 48 hours and warfarin for several weeks except that the dose of warfarin needed to achieve the required reduction of prothrombin activity is likely to be substantially smaller. There is a sound case for the use of I_{125} fibrinogen to detect thrombosis in patients at special risk such as those with stroke or with cardiac failure and this can be a practical policy in a geriatric department (Denham *et al.,* 1973).

Once thromboembolic disease has been diagnosed, treatment should be given automatically except where there are definite contraindications such as recent gastrointestinal bleeding or cerebral haemorrhage or where the patient's condition is considered to be pre-terminal so that further active treatment of any kind would be inappropriate. Recent surgery or cerebral thrombosis do not contraindicate anticoagulant therapy.

Systemic Arterial Embolism

Arterial embolism in the systemic circulation is much less common than pulmonary embolism but may be an equally grave danger. The risks are greatest where the arterial supply to important organs is the site to receive the embolism, for example cerebral, coronary, renal, mesenteric or limb vessel embolism. Apart from subacute bacterial endocarditis, which has been considered elsewhere, major sources of emboli are thrombus in the left auricular appendage in cases of atrial fibrillation, mural cardiac thrombus following myocardial infarction or clot forming in relation to gross atheroma of the aorta or great vessels. Large emboli from this last source may lodge at the aortic bifurcation and lead to bilateral gangrene of the legs, the so-called saddle embolism which carries a very grave prognosis.

17

Diseases of the Gastrointestinal System

There are a number of age changes in the gastro-intestinal tract. These include impairment of taste, deterioration in oesophageal motility, prolongation of gut transit time and a consequent likelihood of developing constipation. In addition, many pathological conditions may commonly affect the elderly.

HIATUS HERNIA

This is very commonly found in old age though it may often be asymptomatic. Women are more often affected and there is an association with obesity.

There are two main types of hiatus hernia, the very common "sliding" type, where the upper part of the stomach and the cardio-oesophageal junction rise up through the diaphragm by direct herniation through the hiatus, and the far less common "rolling" or para-oesophageal type where a portion of the upper stomach herniates through the hiatus alongside the oesophagus so that the cardio-oesophageal junction maintains its normal relationship to the diaphragm. Most of the symptoms of the sliding type are due to interference with the normal "pinch-cock" mechanism exerted upon the cardio-oesophageal junction by the diaphragmatic muscle. In the absence of this, gastric juice can regurgitate into the lower oesophagus where it has considerable irritant effects. Reflux oesophagitis results and if severe may go on to actual peptic ulceration or to stricture formation. The inflammatory changes often result in occult bleeding and when continued lead to iron deficiency anaemia. Indeed hiatus hernia is probably the main cause of iron deficiency anaemia due to blood loss in elderly patients. Reflux oesophagitis gives rise to dyspeptic symptoms of burning epigastric and retrosternal pain accompanied often by flatulence and sometimes by water-brash or acid vomiting. The characteristic feature of the dyspepsia of hiatus hernia of the sliding type is postural aggravation, that is symptoms most often occur in mechanical situations which facilitate regurgitation such as stooping, lying flat or eating a large meal. Patients who sleep with low pillows may be woken up by pain.

Although surgical treatment is available, the results are somewhat questionable and the operation taxing and with a mortality and morbidity which are not negligible. Treatment for elderly patients is thus almost entirely conservative. The main measures are the use of antacids and postural advice to avoid stooping and to sleep with extra pillows or with the head of the bed raised. Obese patients may gain symtomatic relief if they lose weight.

Rolling hiatus hernia is not often seen. Reflux does not occur as the "pinch-cock" mechanism is intact and dyspepsia is usually related to meals.

Hiatus hernia can readily be demonstrated by barium meal examination but in some cases the thoracic part of the stomach may be visible as a shadow behind the heart on the chest X-ray.

PEPTIC ULCER

The clinical features of peptic ulcer are generally little changed in old age and the disease remains quite common even though peak incidence appears to be in middle life. Symptomatology may sometimes be atypical however. Some patients present with non-specific manifestations such as weight loss, general debility, anaemia or painless vomiting.

The occurrence of very large gastric ulcers is not uncommon. In the past it was thought that such "giant" ulcers were often malignant but this is now known to be untrue and most giant ulcers are capable of satisfactory healing which can be surprisingly rapid.

Some peptic ulcers are very chronic ones which first developed in middle life but there are many patients who first get ulcer symptoms in old age. Pulvertaft (1972) has shown that the prognosis for such new ulcers in elderly men is quite good but found that operative mortality, particularly of the Polya type of partial gastrectomy, was disappointingly high. Medical treatment should therefore be thoroughly tried before elective surgical treatment is undertaken and Bilroth type of partial gastrectomy or vagotomy and drainage procedures are to be preferred to the Polya type of operation. Surgical treatment may of course be precipitated by complications. Pyloric obstruction calls for surgical intervention with minimum delay as deterioration may be very rapid with conservative management. Perforation is fortunately not very common in elderly patients but may present very atypically so that diagnosis is delayed with a consequently higher mortality (Coleman & Denham, 1980). Haematemesis is quite common and carries a rather high mortality even when treated promptly.

Cimetidine is now the treatment of choice for acute peptic ulcer in old age. It usually leads to rapid healing of the ulcer though there is a considerable danger of relapse when therapy is discontinued. It has largely supplanted carbenoxolone for, though this is an effective treatment for gastric ulcer, it has troublesome side effects, particularly salt retention and hypokalaemia, and may thus precipitate cardiac failure but the treatment can usefully be employed even in frail old patients provided that careful supervision is maintained. It is known that giving up smoking and bed rest are both capable of assisting ulcer healing. Patients who are smokers should certainly be strongly urged to give up but use of bed rest is probably to be avoided in the old because of its undoubted dangers which are likely to outweigh the possible therapeutic benefit. Ulcer diets are of no proven value and should not be inflicted on the elderly. Antacids can give useful syptomatic relief as may anti-cholinergic drugs but have no influence on ulcer healing. It is important that drugs that may cause gastric irritation, such as aspirin, phenylbutazone or corticosteroids, are carefully avoided.

Effects of Gastric Surgery

Substantial numbers of the elderly, some three percent of the patients admitted to my own department, have had gastric surgery in the past, most commonly Polya type partial gastrectomies. Such operations may result in important late sequelae. Because of reduced gastric capacity, most patients after gastrectomy fail to fully regain their previous usual weight because they eat smaller meals. Some elderly patients are found to be quite severly emaciated as a result of old gastric surgery. In addition gastrectomised patients are liable to various deficiency states, chief of which are iron deficiency anaemia, megaloblastic anaemia and osteomalacia. Iron deficiency anaemia probably results partly from difficulties in absorbing iron but also from losses from occult bleeding from the area of the anastomosis. Megaloblastic anaemia is almost entirely due to B_{12} malabsorption and takes a minimum of four years to become clinically manifest. Osteomalacia is encountered particularly in elderly women, often very many years after their gastric operations, and is probably due to malabsorption of vitamin D coupled with falling exposure to ultra-violet light, which enables vitamin synthesis, as the patient ages and becomes infirm and housebound.

CARCINOMA OF THE STOMACH

The incidence of cancer of the stomach rises with age so that it ranks as one of the commonest malignancies in the elderly. It may present with such non-specific symptoms as weight loss, anorexia, malaise or anaemia, while other cases may show a more characteristic picture with dysphagia, dyspepsia, nausea and vomiting or haematemesis. Some patients may already have advanced disease when they first seek medical advice and may have jaundice, malignant ascites or extensive hepatic or bony metastases.

Diagnosis can usually be readily confirmed by barium meal examination and gastroscopy using a flexible fibroptic endoscope is a useful and practical adjunct permitting the possibility of biopsy confirmation. Many cases are diagnosed at too late a stage for radical surgery to be even considered, but even in cases where it is technically practicable the decision to undertake radical surgery is a dubious one for treatment results are discouragingly poor while operative mortality and morbidity are considerable. It may often prove more realistic to forego the doubtful benefits of radical surgery and either manage the patient conservatively or advise palliative surgery in the form of partial gastrectomy to ameliorate such manifestations as bleeding, dyspepsia or obstructive symptoms.

CARCINOMA OF THE PANCREAS

Pancreatic carcinoma is fairly common in the old. Cases presenting with obstructive jaundice are fairly readily diagnosed but presentation is otherwise likely to be so non-specific as to make recognition a matter of real difficulty, indeed their diagnosis is not rarely first made at post-mortem. The diagnosis should thus be considered when there is an unexplained wasting illness with steady progression. Surgical treatment has nothing to offer the elderly patient with carcinoma of the pancreas other than the palliation of obstructive jaundice.

GALLSTONES

The incidence of gallstones rises with age to the extent that they may be found in up to a third of unselected cases coming to post-mortem. This underlines the fact that in most patients gallstones are totally asymptomatic. Where symptoms do arise, they are closely similar to those in younger age-groups; dyspepsia with fatty intolerance, attacks of cholecystitis or episodes of obstructive jaundice when stones enter the common bile duct. Because asymptomatic stones are so common, the case for surgery when stones are found incidentally is extremely poor. Even when symptoms have occurred, these need to be quite troublesome to justify operation, for cholecystectomy is a fairly major undertaking with appreciable morbidity. On the other hand, when symptoms warrant it, cholecystectomy can be performed successfully even at the most advanced ages.

Because asymptomatic stones occur so commonly, it must be remembered that if gallstones are demonstrated by plain X-ray of abdomen or by cholecystography, this in no way guarantees that they are responsible for the symptoms which prompted investigation.

JAUNDICE IN THE ELDERLY

The differential diagnosis is somewhat modified in old age. Obstructive causes are relatively more common and malignant disease is responsible in a majority. Carcinoma of the pancreas heads the list, obstructing the duct distally, but other carcinomata, especially cancer of the stomach, may produce obstruction more proximally by metastasis to the porta hepatis. Extensive liver metastases may also result in jaundice sometimes although more usually they do not. Gallstones are the other main cause of obstructive jaundice which may show fluctuation in severity while malignant jaundice tends to be steadily progressive. The finding of a palpable gall-bladder is a strong indication that jaundice is due to malignancy for the gall-bladder in cholelithiasis is usually fibrosed as a result of chronic inflammation and thus incapable of distention when the common duct becomes obstructed.

Drug induced jaundice is fairly common and also tends to give an obstructive picture due to intra-hepatic cholestasis. Chlorpromazine is the drug most often responsible but other phenothiazines, anabolic steroids and many other miscellaneous drugs may produce a similar cholestatic picture.

Hepatocellular jaundice is comparatively infrequent. Acute infective hepatitis occurs but is far less common than at earlier ages. Serum hepatitis and cirrhosis, most commonly alcoholic, are other possibilities. Severe jaundice due to haemolysis is rare, but mild jaundice due to pernicious anaemia is quite often seen.

DIVERTICULAR DISEASE OF THE COLON

Diverticular disease becomes very common in older people, post-mortem studies having found prevalences approaching 50 per cent. The findings in diverticular disease are of multiple mucosal herniations arranged in two longitudinal lines at the sites of perforating vessels between the mesenteric tænia and the two lateral tæniae, whose musculature and the circular muscles are hypertrophied. The sigmoid part of the colon is most often involved and the number of diverticula tends to rise with age. Pressure studies have shown that the colon in diverticular disease tends to develop higher intraluminal pressures so that the mucosal herniations are presumably pulsion diverticula.

It has become clear that diverticular disease is rare in more primitive communities and the comparative lack of dietary fibre in the food of more sophisticated populations may be the reason why they suffer a far higher incidence of this condition as a consequence of altered bowel mechanics. A high residue diet, achieved by adding bran as a cheap and acceptable fibre supplement, gives good results in treating patients with diverticular disease giving rise to symptoms.

The very high post-mortem prevalence indicates that diverticular disease remains asymptomatic in the majority of instances. When symptoms develop, these may be abdominal pain, diarrhoea, constipation or alternation of the two and bleeding. Severe complications may arise from the tendency of obstructed diverticula to perforate and thus give rise to peri-colic abscess, peritonitis or fistulae to bladder, vagina or other parts of the gut. Inflammatory masses may form and may result in obstructive symptoms and can closely mimic carcinoma of the colon. Such complications may dictate surgical treatment. Otherwise the medical management comprises the use of a high residue diet to which anti-bacterial therapy may be added, the non-absorbable agents neomycin or phthalylsulphathiazole being common choices.

CARCINOMA OF THE COLON AND RECTUM

Colorectal cancer ranks as the commonest malignancy in those over seventy. Here again there is some evidence to suggest that its high prevalence in the populations of the developed countries may relate to dietary fibre lack (Burkitt, 1971). Despite the fact that about half of colorectal cancers are within range of the examining finger at rectal examination and that about three-quarters are in range of the proctoscope, late diagnosis remains distressingly common. This is particularly unfortunate for surgical treatment of colorectal cancer gives good results with five year survival rates of around 50 per cent and substantially higher rates where the growth has been detected at a pre-symptomatic stage. At the same time, mortality rates for elective surgery are acceptably low. It is therefore important that symptoms such as change in bowel habit, mucous discharge or rectal bleeding should lead to proper investigation, rectal examination being mandatory.

Intestinal obstruction is an important presentation, particularly for growths of the left side of the colon. The less common tumours of the caecum and ascending colon tend to present at a late stage as a large mass in the right iliac fossa, with anaemia or with distant metastases. Large papillary carcinoma of the rectum may result in very severe hypokalaemia because of the secretion of copious, potassium-rich mucous.

DIARRHOEA IN THE ELDERLY

Diarrhoea is a common problem which can present considerable diagnostic difficulties as well as posing a potentially dangerous threat to debilitated, frail patients. Acute diarrhoea often results from dietary indiscretions, particularly from the excessive eating of fruit and especially bananas. Over-enthusiastic use of purgatives is another frequent cause and excessive self-medication with laxatives may explain even long-standing diarrhoea. Spurious diarrhoea is another major cause, most often secondary to faecal impaction but sometimes due to colorectal carcinoma or diverticulitis. Spurious diarrhoea may become quite devastating if heavy purgation is used to alleviate the antecedent constipation. Purgatives should never be prescribed until rectal examination has excluded impaction or other obstruction and where impaction is found, enemata or glycerine suppositories or where necessary manual disimpaction are more correct measures. Drug treatment may produce diarrhoea as a side effect, as is sometimes seen after the use of broad spectrum antibiotics for example. Infective diarrhoea is an important if minor cause of acute diarrhoea. Shigella or Salmonella organisms may be responsible but no bacterial pathogens are found that could account for many minor epidemics of diarrhoea in institutions and these may represent outbreaks due to viral infections or to toxins such as stapylococcal exotoxin.

More persistent diarrhoea may be due to such causes as diverticulitis, occasionally ulcerative colitis and sometimes such miscellaneous conditions as uraemia, thyrotoxicosis, diabetes with autonomic neuropathy, steatorrhoea or gastric and hepatic disease.

18

Diseases of the Central Nervous System

Neurological disease is very common in old age. The high frequency of senile and arteriosclerotic dementia has already been noted. Stroke disease and parkinsonism are also very important causes of disability and the former a major contributor to mortality in old age.

Neurological disease in old age is set against a background of a wide variety of age changes some of which, for example loss of vibration sense and of tendon reflexes in the legs, may modify the interpretation of clinical signs. Other common changes include irregularity and contraction of the pupils and a positive glabellar reflex. There are often deficits of sensory function involving taste, smell, vision and pain perception. Peripheral nerve conduction velocity becomes slowed and autonomic dysfunction is frequently present.

The present chapter will give a highly selective account of central nervous system disease which will concentrate on topics of major clinical importance and on examples of conditions whose natural history is altered in old age.

STROKE AND CEREBROVASCULAR DISEASE

Stroke, a cerebrovascular episode typically of acute onset and resulting in persistent neurological deficit, usually including hemiparesis, is one of the most important medical problems of old age and one which is responsible for very heavy demands on health services as well as being a major cause of death in the age group.

Although the common underlying pathology is basically the same, that is atherosclerosis, the actual mechanism resulting in a stroke may be considered under the three main headings of cerebral thrombosis, cerebral haemorrhage and cerebral embolism. However in individual cases the recognition of the precise mechanism may be a difficult and essentially academic exercise. Certainly some strokes result from occlusion of extra-cerebral vessels such as the carotid or vertebral arteries or they may follow a sudden fall in cardiac output which lowers cerebral perfusion and leads to non-occlusive infarction in such circumstances as acute myocardial infarction, massive pulmonary embolism or haemorrhagic shock.

Clinically, stroke may pass through different phases and one may speak of "completed stroke" or of "stroke in evolution" or "ingravescent stroke". In other cases a stroke may rapidly exhibit complete recovery and such episodes, particularly when repeated, are referred to as "transient ischaemic attacks".

Cerebral Thrombosis. Cerebral thrombosis is probably the main cause of stroke in the elderly although many cases so diagnosed may in fact have no clear evidence of thrombosis at post-mortem examination and are perhaps more correctly examples of non-occlusive infarction resulting from a combination of vascular narrowing and transient haemodynamic changes. Cerebrovascular accidents due to cerebral thrombosis typically have a moderately rapid onset, hemiparesis or other neurological deficit coming on over the course of some minutes or even hours. Coma ensues in only a minority of cases, many having no disturbance of consciousness or merely becoming drowsy. It is not rare for the stroke to come on during sleep so that the patient awakes with a completed stroke. A few cases may however show the picture of ingravescent stroke with progressive increase of signs over several days. Others again may have brief episodes of premonitory symptoms in the days immediately before the stroke, consisting of such manifestations as transient giddiness, dysarthria, dysphasia, confusion, limb weakness or paraesthesiae.

Cerebral Haemorrhage. Cerebral haemorrhage is less common than thrombosis. It is more likely to be associated with hypertension and it carries a very much worse prognosis. Indeed most deaths in the first few days after a stroke are accounted for by cases of cerebral haemorrhage whilst they form quite a small proportion of long-term survivors from stroke. Haemorrhage may be purely subarachnoid but in such cases is usually from rupture of an atherosclerotic vessel and rarely from a congenital aneurism. More often the vascular rupture is intra-cerebral but if sufficiently disruptive may break out into the subarachnoid space to produce bloodstained cerebro-spinal fluid.

The typical stroke due to haemorrhage has a sudden and dramatic onset which may be heralded by headache or vomiting. Rapidly deepening disturbance of consciousness is frequent and neck stiffness may be found when bleeding into the cerebro-spinal fluid has taken place. Severe cases may develop papilloedema and neurological signs may become bilateral because of gross midline shift. Deep coma may lead to very early death.

Cerebral Embolism. Cerebral embolism is responsible for perhaps five or ten percent of strokes in the elderly. Here onset is virtually instantaneous, that is there is immediately a complete stroke and any change after that is one of improvement. Important sources of emboli are thrombus in the left auricular appendage, especially in association with mitral valve disease and auricular fibrillation, and cardiac mural thrombus following acute myocardial infarction. There is always a risk of repeated embolism leading to a succession of strokes but apart from this special risk, the general prognosis of embolic strokes is superior to that of cerebral haemorrhage although rather less favourable than that for thrombosis. Coma in cerebral embolism is seldom deep or prolonged.

Management of Stroke. Prognosis of stroke can perhaps best be gauged by the duration and the severity of disturbance of consciousness. Mortality is very high indeed if patients remain in coma for over 24 hours. Comatose patients, who as we have already noted are usually examples of stroke due to cerebral haemorrhage, require careful nursing care with particular attention being paid to the prevention of pressure sores by frequent turning and to maintaining an airway. Pharyngeal aspiration with a sucker is usually necessary to keep it clear of secretions and catheterisation is advisable. Fluids should only be given by nasogastric tube in comatose stroke patients when the outlook for recovery is reasonably favourable. Hypostatic pneumonia is a common and often lethal complication but there is no evidence that prophylactic administration of antibiotics can help to prevent it. Indeed antibiotics are probably disadvantageous as they may merely ensure that the infection is with resistant organisms when it comes. Management is essentially conservative and heroic measures such as tracheostomy or resuscitation for cardiac arrest can seldom by justifiable. There is no reason to believe that special measures such as carbon dioxide inhalation, corticosteroid therapy or stellate ganglion block confer any advantage. Surgical intervention may sometimes be worth considering where there is deepening unconsciousness due to an expanding intracerebral haematoma. Clot evacuation can sometimes result in significant improvement.

If impaired consciousness persists, regular extension of joints to prevent the development of contractures needs to be started and should of course be continued throughout a patient's rehabilitation in the case of the paralysed limbs.

Rehabilitation proper should commence as soon as the patient regains consciousness or immediately following the stroke in the many patients in whom consciousness was never affected. There is nothing to show that an initial period of rest should be interposed and indeed there are many reasons to suppose that such a period of inactivity may well be detrimental. For example, balance is often a key factor which may limit rehabilitation progress and it seems that this deteriorates very rapidly if there is a period of recumbency. Postural hypotension, a common problem after stroke, is also made worse by recumbency and this is also the case for venous thrombosis. This last complication is particularly relevant for pulmonary embolism from deep vein thrombosis is the main cause of death within the early weeks for patients with stroke who have survived the first few days during which deaths related to the stroke itself occur. Unfortunately these thromboembolic deaths are by no means prevented by a policy of early mobilisation and the risk is high during the first ten to fourteen days particularly. Finally bed rest favours the development of hypostatic pneumonia, another potentially lethal complication.

Once the first fortnight has been successfully negotiated, the subsequent prognosis for life in stroke patients is quite good. Furthermore, the prognosis for successful rehabilitation is by no means gloomy as Adams (1971) describes. There is thus a case for reasonable optimism in the management of stroke patients and treatment should thus be prompt, energetic and applied with both enthusiasm and persistence. Whilst early improvement implies a more favourable prognosis, its absence must not lead to the premature discontinuation of active treatment for there are a significant number of patients who may show no signs of improvement for many weeks or even some months and yet may ultimately make a useful recovery. In some such patients rehabilitation may take up to a year or even longer and yet they may in the end recover to an extent that allows them to return home to a life of reasonable independence.

Anticoagulant treatment plays no regular part in the treatment of completed stroke except when venous thrombosis or pulmonary embolism have occured as complications. Cerebral embolism is an exception to this generalisation however and calls for anticoagulant therapy which should be continued for some months at least. Stroke patients who are hypertensive and who have survived the initial danger period of the acute stage of the illness seem to have a prognosis that is no worse, and may indeed be even marginally better, than normotensive patients with stroke. There is thus no case for treatment of their hypertension unless this is indicated on other grounds such as coexistent heart failure.

Rehabilitation of the Stroke Patient. The reasons for starting rehabilitation promptly have already been enumerated. Because balance can so readily deteriorate, great efforts should be made to prevent such loss and, where limb weakness prevents weight bearing, a start can be made by practising balance in the sitting position or with the knee temporarily splinted the patient may practise standing balance with assistance. Where leg power is sufficient, standing balance should be started and, once this is adequate, walking practice should commence. The patient should also practise rising from a chair using the technique described in Chapter 8.

Occupational therapy is of great importance in the re-education of hand function as well as in the reacquisition of important practical skills such as washing, dressing and cooking. New techniques and gadgets and devices may allow successful performance of such necessary activities of daily living even when hand recovery is so poor that the patient becomes one handed in functional terms.

Barriers to Recovery. Apart from such general barriers to recovery as associated pre-existing disabilities, poor exercise tolerance or poor morale and motivation, the stroke itself may give rise to more specific obstacles and Adams (1971) has done much to clarify these. A major group are associated neurological disabilities other than the hemiplegia itself. Perhaps the most important of all these is the major intellectual deficit which may follow the stroke. Indeed the small proportion of stroke survivors who cannot be rehabilitated and become long-stay patients are nearly all moderately or severely demented, may have poor concentration and motivation and are usually incontinent. Next in seriousness is dysphasia and dysphasic strokes too make a significant contribution to the geriatric long-stay patient population. Other important barriers to recovery are sensory disturbances, hemianopia, ataxia and various agnosias.

Depression is a not uncommon consequence of severe stroke, particularly when dysphasia is present. This can greatly hinder successful rehabilitation and may often be a sufficient problem to justify treatment with tricyclic antidepressants.

Dysphasia. Dysphasia occurs in a substantial minority of strokes in old age, usually in association with right hemiplegia but sometimes as an isolated finding with no limb weakness at all. Dysphasia needs to be clearly distinguished from mental confusion and the two are most likely to be mistaken when there is "jargon" dysphasia; a form of dysphasia when considerable sensory aphasia is accompanied by bizarre speech with many neologisms so that the talk may sound completely "mad". Almost total aphasia also needs to be distinguished from anarthria or aphonia. Detailed discussion of dysphasia is beyond our present scope and the reader is referred to standard textbooks.

Dysphasia represents perhaps one of the most terrible catastrophes that may befall patients. Its sudden onset thus often leads to considerable emotional disturbance. The precipitation of depression has already been noted but others may become anxious or emotionally labile. In men particularly, the intense frustration engendered by dysphasia may lead to aggressive behaviour and outbursts of bad temper which require sensitive and sympathetic handling. Indeed much of the help speech therapists may give to dysphasic patients is perhaps in the alleviation of their emotional responses to the disability rather than in terms of actual improvement in the disability itself. Those looking after the dysphasic need to give him opportunity to practise his remaining speech skills and must therefore be prepared to listen patiently and to speak back intelligently and not as if to some kind of halfwit. They should not forget that patients with severe motor dysphasia may none the less have retained good comprehension and should be careful not to make tactless remarks in their hearing, assuming that these cannot be understood.

Transient Ischaemic Attacks. Transient ischaemic attacks are an interesting if not particularly common phenomenon in the old. Their incidence is often overstated and episodes of epilepsy, Stokes-Adams attacks or postural hypotension are all too likely to be wrongly accorded this rather trendy diagnosis.

Transient ischaemic attacks are believed to be due to arterial disease in either the carotid or the vertebro-basilar systems and consist of episodes recovering fully within 24 hours in which a variety of disturbances of cerebral function may occur such as giddiness, true vertigo, occular symptoms or transient speech disturbance or limb paresis. There is some evidence from ophthalmoscopic observations during such attacks that multiple platelet emboli may be responsible. These presumably originate from thrombi based on atheromatous plaques in the major artery supplying the involved area.

The tendency to over-diagnose transient ischaemic attacks has been alluded to and the diagnosis should not be indiscriminately applied to minor episodes of giddiness and suchlike. Neither should falls in old people be given the alluring name of "drop attacks" and uncritically ascribed to vertebro-basilar insufficiency. Where the diagnosis of transient ischaemic attacks can be substantiated, long term anticoagulant therapy should be seriously considered for there is a not inconsiderable risk of subsequent development of a completed stroke.

Sub-dural Haematoma. Sub-dural haematoma is important as a condition of relatively frequent occurrence which is amenable to surgical treatment. It typically develops after injury to the head but this need only be minor and the clinical picture may take some weeks to become manifest. A characteristic feature is fluctuating drowsiness and confusion which may or may not be accompanied by focal neurological signs and uncommonly by consequences of raised intracranial pressure such as headache, vomiting and papilloedema. Skull X-ray may show midline shift and brain scans may show typical peripheral areas of increased uptake. Computerised axial tomography (C.A.T. scan) will often clinch the diagnosis. Reasonable suspicion of a sub-dural haematoma should lead to prompt neurosurgical referral. Surgical treatment consists of making of burr holes and evacuation of the clot which is not uncommonly bilateral. Results can be most gratifying but it must be admitted that they are substantially less good than in younger patients. Some patients are left with permanent intellectual impairment or focal signs and there is a significant mortality. None the less, the potential benefits of surgery are such that every effort should be made to ensure that the diagnosis is not overlooked.

Cerebral Tumour. Although cerebral secondary deposits, particularly from adenocarcinoma of lung, account for a substantial minority of cases of cerebral tumours in old age, primary cerebral tumour is not rare. Meningioma is quite common and quite a number are found as incidental findings at post-mortem. Others however may give rise to symptoms of space occupation with a very slowly progressive clinical course. Glioma is almost equally common. These have a far more rapid clinical course, often presenting with progressive hemiplegia, confusion or dysphasia. Vomiting, headache and papilloedema may be late in appearing. Stroke may be more closely simulated when haemorrhage into the tumour leads to the sudden onset of hemiplegia but the subsequent insidious deterioration may give the clue to the true diagnosis. C.A.T. and isotope scans are useful and safe but the dangers of lumbar puncture should be remembered and the test omitted where tumour seems a likely diagnosis because of the risk of precipitating fatal coning of the medulla. Unfortunately surgical intervention is of little or no value in elderly patients with glioma but can be well worthwhile in meningioma. Dexamethasone therapy may result in useful if temporary remission quite often in patients with glioma and is usually worth a try.

PARKINSON'S DISEASE

In old age, parkinsonism is of considerable importance because of its very high prevalence, about 10 per cent in admissions to geriatric departments, and because reasonably effective treatment is available.

The clinical picture is considerably modified in old age. The most striking difference is that tremor, often the most prominent feature in middle-aged patients, is often unobtrusive or may even be totally absent so that rigidity is the major manifestation of the syndrome. Another important difference is that associated mental impairment is quite common and may be very severe. This is in contrast to experience in younger subjects where mental impairment is uncommon, although perhaps not as rare as was implied by much of the older literature.

The aetiology of parkinsonism in old age is often uncertain. Post-encephalitic parkinsonism is now rare and drug-induced parkinsonism accounts for only a small proportion of cases. The remaining bulk of cases have often been labelled "arteriosclerotic parkinsonism", however there is no real evidence that they are in fact due to arteriosclerosis as such patients show no excess of arteriosclerotic disease elsewhere and post-mortem studies fail to demonstrate any clear contribution by vascular changes to the diffuse extra-pyramidal damage which is to be found. The majority of cases are thus of unknown cause but perhaps should not be termed "idiopathic parkinsonism" as this term is applied to the "paralysis agitans" group of cases who typically have an onset in late middle life and have tremor as a prominent feature and are thus clinically a very different group. The natural history of parkinsonism in old age is quite variable, suggesting that a variety of aetiologies may underlie the syndrome. An important clinical variant is where dementia is the most striking facet of the clinical picture and where progression is typically rapid. At the other extreme there are many mild cases of parkinsonism with little or no mental impairment in whom progression may be very slow.

Diagnosis of Parkinsonism. Recognition of a typical case, particularly where tremor is obvious, presents little difficulty but cases of parkinsonism where tremor is inconspicuous may easily be overlooked even when rigidity is gross and responsible for significant disability. In such patients, the characteristic facies with fixed expression and infrequent blinking and stare is a useful pointer. Abnormalities of gait such as small pace, reduced arm swing, bent posture and tendency to propulsion, may be useful in drawing attention to the possibility of the diagnosis. Voice changes can be similarly of value, the typical change being monotonous tone coupled with poor volume. The finding of rigidity is the main confirmatory sign when tremor is absent. Even in the absence of obvious tremor, limb rigidity may show the cogwheel phenomenon. Where limb tone is difficult to assess because of poor cooperation. Wartenberg's head drop test (Chapter 4) can be of special value, particularly as neck rigidity tends to appear early in the development of parkinsonism. The glabella reflex, the persistence of blinking in response to repeated tapping just above the junction of the eyebrows, although almost always positive in parkinsonism, is of little diagnostic value as it is so often positive in other old people, especially those with other types of diffuse cerebral damage.

Consequences of Parkinsonism. Parkinsonism commonly leads to increasing immobility, and to particularly difficulty in rising from a chair and moving in bed. Clumsiness of the hands and impairment of fine movement leading for example to deterioration in handwriting, which becomes cramped and small, is frequent. Patients are highly susceptible to falls and these may be both frequent and severe. They presumably relate to the stiffness and slowness of movement so that, once threatened, balance cannot be regained in time to avoid a fall. There is also a special risk of the development of pressure sores, particularly heel sores, and these may occur even in ambulant patients who are constitutionally well because of their specific difficulty in moving freely in bed. This risk needs to be clearly recognised and a bed cradle is a simple aid to prevention as it makes movement in bed considerably easier.

Treatment of Parkinsonism. When parkinsonism results in significant disability which can be ascribed to rigidity, weakness or bradykinesis of the muscles, treatment is indicated. Treatment should not be given purely because the diagnosis of parkinsonism has been made for all forms of drug treatment of the disease have troublesome side effects and treatment can only affect the symptoms and not the underlying progression of the disease.

All drug therapy is effective against rigidity and associated weakness and bradykinesia but has little or no effect on tremor. This is seldom a snag in the elderly where tremor is usually an insignificant problem. The earliest effective drugs were the belladonna alkaloids introduced by Charcot. Later, a group of more effective drugs were synthesized which were related to atropine and remained the drugs of choice for many years. Benzhexol (artane) and orphenadrine (disipal) were the most widely used of these drugs. However, atropine-like antiparkinsonian drugs only have a very incomplete therapeutic effect and even this is obtained at a considerable risk of toxic effects. Mental confusion is chief among these and was particularly associated with the use of benzhexol in elderly patients. Other side effects are atropine-like, for example drying of the mouth, blurred vision and retention of urine. Now that other drugs are available there is no place for benzhexol in the treatment of

Parkinson's disease in old age though the other less toxic atropine-like drugs may still have a limited role.

Two important new drugs were introduced in the sixties and have rendered the atropine-like drugs largely obsolescent. These are L dopa and amantidine. Amantidine is not greatly used in the elderly as it is less powerful than L dopa, may give serious confusional states often marked by gross visual hallucinosis and because its effects may weaken after several weeks in some patients. L dopa, in contrast, has proved to be one of the most important advances in the treatment of elderly patients of recent years. Whe first introduced L dopa was used alone, the dose being built up in 500 mg steps to a maximum tolerated dosage of usually 2-3 grams per day. However, though a very effective drug, side effects were a considerable problem which often made it impossible to give a sufficient dose to achieve optimum therapeutic benefit. Most troublesome toxic effects comprised nausea, vomiting and other gastrointestinal symptoms.

L dopa is now usually given in combination with a dopa decarboxylase inhibitor which does not cross the blood-brain barrier. This reduces the peripheral metabolism of L dopa so that its central effects are increased approximately five-fold. The smaller effective dose reduces peripheral side effects, particularly nausea and vomiting, though not influenceing the central side effects of mental disturbance, postural hypotension and dyskinetic syndromes. These combined preparations (sinemet and madopar) are now the treatment of choice in elderly patients with Parkinson's disease. However when L dopa preparations are poorly tolerated or fail to achieve sufficient clinical benefit, amantadine or drugs of the atropine group can be added to the treatment regime and have additive effects. However toxic effects are very likely to occur in such complex regimes and when they do it may be hard to tell which drug is to blame and therefore to decide which to withdraw.

Surgical treatment of parkinsonism is rarely justified in elderly patients. Even in younger patients its use has declined since the advent of L dopa and this drug is almost always given a thorough trial before surgery is now considered.

Chorea

Mild cases of chorea are seen regularly in old people. It is not clear whether the aetiology is arteriosclerotic or degenerative and the noncommittal term "senile chorea" is often employed. In some of the cases the choreiform movements of the limbs are of sufficient degree to interfere with walking and balance. Such patients may be helped by drug therapy, phenothiazines such as perphenazine (fentazin) which have marked parkinsonian side effects being capable of effectively damping down the troublesome involuntary movements. Tetrabenazine may also be useful.

Peripheral Neuritis

In old age, peripheral neuritis may arise from a bewildering variety of causes. Chief among these are diabetic neuropathy and the neuropathy occuring in association with carcinoma, especially bronchial cancer. Drug toxicity, for example from furadantin, ischaemic neuropathy and peripheral neuritis due to rheumatoid arthritis are other important possibilities. As in other age-groups, a substantial proportion of cases of peripheral neuritis cannot be ascribed to any recognisable cause.

Motor Neurone Disease

More motor neurone disease is seen in old age than textbook accounts of the disease would suggest. Furthermore its prognosis is far better in many old patients than is commonly allowed. It is not rare to see survivals of over ten years even where there is bulbar involvement and I have seen several cases with survivals of near twenty years (Hodkinson, 1972).

Cervical Spondylosis

Degenerative disease of the spine is virtually ubiquitous in old age. The mere finding of advanced cervical spondylosis on X-ray is thus quite commonplace and should not be taken as proof that neurological changes present are due to cervical spondylosis. In fact neurological consequences of cervical spondylosis seem to be a considerable rarity in old age both in regard to myelopathy and to the brachalgia syndrome. Myelopathy more commonly proves to be due to carcinoma, diabetes or subacute combined degeneration of the cord.

Autonomic Dysfunction

Impairment of autonomic function is now known to be a common feature of old age (see review by Exton-Smith, 1978). Autonomic neuropathy may accompany peripheral neuropathy, particularly in diabetes. Autonomic dysfunction may be associated with, for example, Parkinson's disease or Shy-Drager syndrome. In many elderly patients however autonomic dysfunction has no ready explanation and may represent a change due to ageing.

The practical consequences of autonomic dysfunction are chiefly postural hypotension (chapter 16) and hypothermia (chapter 6), both of which are important clinical problems in elderly patients.

Herpes Zoster

This troublesome condition rises in frequency with age. Pain in the distribution of the affected nerve root may precede the occurrence of the rash and cause considerable diagnostic confusion. However the diagnosis should be obvious once the rash appears. Shingles may result in considerable constitutional upset and the eye complications of the common ophthalmic herpes zoster often call for careful treatment in hospital. The persistence of root pain as post-herpetic neuralgia is unfortunately all too common in old age. This can be a disheartening condition to treat, simple analgesics being the mainstay but depression may result from the disabling complaint and call for antidepressant therapy on occasions. Treatment of acute herpes zoster with corticosteroids has been claimed to result in a diminished incidence of subsequent post-herpetic neuralgia but this remains an unproven assertion. In view of the major side effects of steroids it is difficult to recommend their use in this situation.

Further Reading

Adams, G F (1974) Cerebrovascular disability and the ageing brain, Churchill Livingstone, Edinburgh.
Hildick-Smith, M (1980) Management of Parkinson's disease in the elderly, p 215-258 in The treatment of medical problems in the elderly, Ed. Denham, M J, MTP Press, Lancaster.

19

Diseases of the Kidney and Uro-genital System

Renal function shows gradual and progressive changes with age. The kidneys become smaller in size and the nephrons become less in size and number. Basement membranes thicken and the arterial tree atrophies. In functional terms there is a comparable deterioration with elevation of blood urea and decline of glomerular filtration rate. Tubular efficiency also falls as shown by tests of tubular secretion and of concentration and dilution. This falling functional capacity of the kidney with age means that the elderly have less of a reserve of renal function and are correspondingly vulnerable to the effects of disease. Uraemia is thus a common clinical situation.

URAEMIA

Even in normal old people, the range for blood urea is somewhat higher than in earlier age-groups (3.9-9.9 mmol/l cf 3.5-7.2 for younger adults). In ill old people modest elevation of urea beyond these levels is a very common finding and may not require any special action or further investigation. Similar changes are seen in serum creatinine values except that where lean body mass is much reduced they may be unexpectedly low. Even when serum creatinine values are corrected for such changes in body mass they have been shown to be marginally less good than blood urea as a guide to the glomerular filtration rate of elderly patients (Denham *et al.*, 1975). Substantial degrees of renal impairment are, however, quite commonly found in elderly patients and such uraemia can be considered under three main groupings.

Pre-renal Uraemia

Pre-renal uraemia is overwhelmingly the most frequent situation in the aged. It is due to a fall in renal blood flow leading to a fall in glomerular filtration rate sufficient to impair renal function and result in nitrogen retention. The chief cause in ill old people is dehydration which may develop from a simple failure to drink adequately or may be aggravated by such factors as diarrhoea, vomiting or over-treatment with diuretics. Pre-renal uraemia may also result when cardiac output falls in such conditions as haemorrhagic shock, acute myocardial infarction or heart failure.

Pre-renal uraemia may result in very high urea levels even when there is no associated structural renal disease. Despite common statements to the contrary, serum creatinine tends to rise *pari passu* with urea in the elderly with pre-renal uraemia and so does not help in distinguishing it from renal uraemia. Serum bicarbonate may however be of value for this is normal in pre-renal uraemia but is typically low in renal uraemia.

The prompt and correct recognition of pre-renal uraemia is of considerable importance as, with treatment of the underlying cause, it is potentially completely reversible. Recognition of dehydration is of special relevance and serum urea and electrolytes are indispensable routine investigations in the ill elderly patient.

Post-renal Uraemia

Post-renal uraemia results when there is obstruction of urinary outflow from the kidneys so that renal function is impaired by a back-pressure effect. Although less common than pre-renal uraemia it is equally important as a potentially reversible cause of uraemia. Recognition needs to be prompt for sustained back-pressure can lead to irreversible renal damage. Common causes of post-renal uraemia are obstruction by benign prostatic hypertrophy, carcinoma of the prostate and carcinoma of the bladder.

Renal Uraemia

There remain those cases of uraemia that are due to disease of the kidney itself and included among them may be many instances of irreversible and progressive renal decompensation. Acute renal failure may occur from a variety of renal pathologies but is not very common and is essentially similar to acute renal failure in younger age-groups and will not be considered further. Chronic renal failure is relatively common with chronic pyelonephritis as its principal cause. Renal failure due to hypertension is infrequent as is that due to diabetic nephropathy, a somewhat surprising situation as diabetes is so common in the age-group. Chronic glomerulonephritis is uncommon and acute glomerulonephritis a considerable rarity whilst nephrotic syndrome is infrequent.

Chronic Renal Failure

The clinical picture of chronic renal failure in old age is broadly similar to that in middle life. However there are differences of detail in that mental confusion is more often seen whilst headache is an uncommon symptom. General deterioration, wasting, nausea and drowsiness are important mani-festations and hiccough, diarrhoea or gastro-intestinal bleeding may be seen in advanced cases. Some degree of anaemia commonly develops and acidosis with a low serum bicarbonate is frequent. Sodium depletion is not un-common and is of special importance as it may lead to further deterioration of renal function.

Management of Renal Failure

The importance of the correct recognition and prompt treatment of pre-renal or post-renal factors has already been stressed and these may of course coexist in patients with renal uraemia. The management of chronic renal failure is otherwise largely conservative for renal transplantation or chronic dialysis are hardly ever justifiable in old age. In the common situation where chronic pyelonephritis is the underlying cause, the control of renal infection is important but calls for special care in the choice of antibiotics as those excreted by the kidney will reach very high and often toxic blood levels.

An important general measure is the encouragement of an increased fluid intake. This will deal with any unrecognised pre-renal element due to dehydration but also allows the isosthenuric kidney to excrete to the maximum possible by producing more urine of relatively fixed composition. Acidosis should be corrected by administration of sodium bicarbonate or sodium citrate and if sodium depletion is present this calls for sodium chloride supplementation but over-treatment leading to the precipitation of heart failure must be avoided. Potassium containing medicines must be used with special care as potassium retention is an important and potentially lethal feature of renal failure.

Uraemia can be partially controlled by reducing protein intake while ensuring a good calorie intake to prevent unnecessary protein catabolism. Special diets with low protein and high carboydrate are not very pleasant and are a considerable imposition upon the elderly uraemic patient. Their use needs careful consideration for we need to be sure that they make the patient's existence more tolerable and not the reverse.

It is usually of little help to actively treat the anaemia which usually results from chronic uraemia. Haematinics seldom have any effect and transfusion usually results in only a very short-lived rise in the haemoglobin level and in view of its hazards is not generally advisable.

URINARY TRACT INFECTION

Urinary tract infection is an important problem in old age. Many workers have reported high incidences of significant bacteriuria in the elderly in the community and more particularly in elderly hospital patients. The bacteriuria is most often asymptomatic but may be associated with mild dysuria or frequency especially in females. It is an open question as to whether asymptomatic significant bacteriuria should be treated and actively looked for. The very high reported incidences make it a daunting proposal, particularly as obtaining reliable urine specimens presents very considerable practical difficulties. The ordinary mid-stream specimen of urine is highly fallible unless taken with obsessional care in a fully cooperative patient and urinary aspiration by needle puncture of the distended bladder, though a valuable and safe technique, calls for good patient cooperation and is difficult to do as a routine. At the present time most geriatricians do not routinely search for and treat asymptomatic bacteriuria but there is room for a range of opinion in the matter, the opposing views being usefully reviewed by Sourander (1978).

Cystitis

Mechanical or neurological factors which lead to urinary stasis in the bladder favour the development of infection. Thus cystitis may occur in association with such conditions as benign prostatic hypertrophy, bladder diverticula, bladder stone or abnormalities of neurological control of the bladder as in paraplegia or in the irritable bladder of arteriosclerotic or senile dementia. Additional factors are the short urethra in the female which makes bacterial invasion relatively easier and catheterisation or other instrumentation of the bladder.

Cystitis may give frequency, burning dysuria and pain over the bladder and may sometimes produce fever and constitutional upset. In other cases however the symptoms may be quite unobtrusive and persistent urinary infection go unheeded.

Pyelonephritis

Pyelonephritis is a more serious form of urinary tract infection and when chronic can lead to permanent structural damage of the kidneys resulting in chronic renal failure. Acute attacks of pyelonephritis may present as in middle life with loin pain, fever, rigors and severe constitutional upset but rather more commonly the picture is a less dramatic one. Confusional states are not uncommonly due to acute pyelonephritis. Chronic pyelonephritis may be an essentially asymptomatic condition although sometimes punctuated by acute exacerbations. Finally however it will tend to result in uraemia and progressive chronic renal failure.

Treatment of Urinary Tract Infection

Because of the importance of pyelonephritis in the aetiology of chronic renal failure, urinary infection in old age needs to be seriously regarded. Bacteriological examination of carefully obtained mid-stream urinary specimens should be a common if not routine investigation and where significant bacteriuria and pyuria exist or where significant bacteriuria accompanies urinary symptoms or chronic renal failure, treatment is definitely indicated.

Treatment is favoured by a good fluid intake and this should be strongly encouraged. The commonest infecting organism is *E. coli* so that amoxycillin or cotrimoxazole are often appropriate choices as chemotherapy. Choice will of course be influenced by the results of bacteriological culture and sensitivity tests. Nitrofurantoin and nalidixic acid are useful drugs but their excretion in the urine is very poor in renal failure. Tetracyclines are contraindicated in renal failure as they may result in rising urea levels.

Generally, 5-7 days of chemotherapy may be indicated but in chronic pyelonephritis there is a case for prolonged treatment. Because of problems of the emergence of bacterial resistance, especially when multiple organisms are involved, the urinary antiseptic hexamine mandelate (mandelamine) can be usefully employed and is to be preferred to the rotational use of antibiotics. Mandelamine is one of the least toxic agents available and its action is enhanced by acidification of the urine. Ascorbic acid (three or more half-gram tablets daily) can be used for this purpose.

PROSTATIC DISEASE

Benign Prostatic Hypertrophy

Benign prostatic hypertrophy is very common in old men. When it leads to dysuria, typically with frequency, poor stream, dribbling and nocturia, or results in acute retention or chronic retention with overflow, the treatment is primarily surgical. The standard operation of retropubic prostatectomy has been brought to a very high level of safety in old age so that it can be offered to all but the most decrepid old men. Even where the risk is thought too great, the less taxing operation of per-urethral resection can be utilised and the recent introduction of cryosurgery of the prostate may prove to offer an even smaller operative risk. Thus only a very occasional patient with complications of benign prostatic hypertrophy should need to be condemned to a permanent catheter life and the miseries and risks which it entails.

Carcinoma of the Prostate

This is the most frequent neoplasm in elderly men. Indeed carcinoma *in situ* can be found in amazingly high proportions of prostates of old men at post-mortem although the relationship of such histological findings to clinical carcinoma of prostate is not clear. Presentation of carcinoma of prostate is sometimes with dysuria or urinary retention but rather more often occurs because of secondary spread. Bone secondaries are particularly common and give rise to skeletal pain. The metastases are usually osteo-sclerotic, this appearance, although not pathognomonic, being a strong pointer to the diagnosis. Rectal examination will typically show a hard and irregular prostate which may not be particularly large. Previous prostatectomy does not preclude the development of carcinoma of the prostate.

When the cancer presents with obstructive symptoms or retention, surgical treatment is usually needed. Where metastasis has occurred the serum acid phosphatase is often raised and can be a useful diagnostic test. Treatment of metastatic disease is with oestrogens and results can be very gratifying, remissions of several years in cases with advanced bone metastasis being far from uncommon. Stilboestrol is the drug most often used. This can result in side effects of nausea and troublesome sodium retention leading to cardiac failure though these problems are less common now it has been recognised that there is no advantage in giving larger doses of stilboestrol, 1 mg/day being sufficient for a full therapeutic effect.

GYNAECOLOGICAL DISORDERS

A wide range of gynaecological disorders may be encountered in old age and have been usefully reviewed by Brown (1978). A common problem which is particular to postmenopausal women is atrophic or 'senile' vaginitis. This represents atrophy of the vaginal epithelium consequent upon the lowering of oestrogen levels after the menopause. Furthermore, there are changes in the vaginal flora so that secretions loose the acidity which protects the vagina from infection in younger women. Secondary infection is thus far more likely and elderly women may complain of pain, pruritus or of discharge which may be bloodstained. The condition responds well to oestrogens given either orally or locally as creams.

20

Endocrine Disease

While many endocrine diseases may be seen occasionally in old age, three conditions stand out in importance because of their frequency, diabetes, thyrotoxicosis and myxoedema. The present account will concentrate on these three but will also consider hyperparathyroidism more briefly. Other endocrine diseases, and particularly disorders of the hypophyso-adrenal axis, are distinctly uncommon in old age.

DIABETES MELLITUS

Diabetes is extremely common in old age by any criteria. The criteria do indeed pose some difficulties for high blood sugar and abnormalities of the glucose tolerance test are common in old age and are taken by some as evidence of the very high incidence of diabetes while others suggest because of their frequency that more lax standards of normality should be applied in the elderly. However there is no sound evidence to support this last view and it seems wiser to apply the same standards to the old as to the young in interpreting glucose tolerance tests and blood sugar results.

Diabetes in the elderly is often mild and most cases have their onset in old age. Clinical cases, that is those with symptoms or complications attributable to diabetes, are outnumbered by asymptomatic cases which may be discovered by routine blood sugar determinations or by the finding of glycosuria. Random blood sugar is in fact a far more effective screening test than glycosuria as the latter may not develop even with a considerably raised blood sugar level because renal threshold for glucose is commonly elevated in the elderly. Furthermore random blood sugar is effective in the detection of diabetes, fasting blood sugars being unnecessary as well as inconvenient. Routine random blood sugar should certainly be a part of the investigation of all elderly patients admitted to hospital.

Many cases of diabetes in the elderly occur in association with obesity. Very occasional cases may prove to be associated with pancreatic disease and the rapid onset of severe diabetes may be the mode of presentation in carcinoma of the pancreas. Diabetes may also be precipitated by the use of thiazide diuretics in predisposed subjects. Corticosteroid therapy may be similarly responsible.

Symptoms and Complications of Diabetes

Thirst and polyuria are important symptoms and severe wasting may occur in some patients although patients are more often obese. Pruritis vulvae is sometimes a pointer to the diagnosis. Very often however diabetes is found incidentally or because it has presented with a complication of the disease. Vascular complications are particularly common. Retinopathy may lead to visual impairment and where microaneurisms or typical waxy exudates are present, ophthalmoscopic appearances are practically diagnostic. Peripheral vascular disease is also a serious complication which may present with gangrene or, when peripheral neuropathy is also present, with penetrating ulceration of the foot often accompanied by chronic osteomyelitis of the bones of the foot. Both stroke and ischaemic heart disease are more common in diabetes because of the association of atherosclerosis. Neuropathy is another important complication and is most often seen as a predominantly sensory polyneuritis affecting the legs which is capable of improvement with control of the underlying diabetes. Alternatively, autonomic neuropathy may occur and may be manifested by postural hypotension or by nocturnal diarrhoea. Diabetic nephropathy of the Kimmelsteil-Wilson type is not very common but as pyelonephritis is common in association with diabetes, renal failure is not a rare complication. Cataract is more common in the elderly with diabetes than in those without although the diabetic and senile cataract are indistinguishable.

Treatment of Diabetes

Mild late onset diabetes, often associated with obesity, can often be controlled simply by adequate dietary restriction of carbohydrate to around 100 G/day. This accounts for a majority of cases but substantial numbers will need oral treatment to be added to the dietary regime. The sulphonylureas tolbutamide, chlorpropamide and glibenclamide are the most useful drugs though the biguanide metformin may be added if the suphonylurea fails to give adequate control. All the sulphonylurea drugs carry the risk of precipitating hypoglycaemic attacks and the long acting chlorpropamide is particularly likely to give trouble.

If hyperglycaemia cannot be controlled by the combination of diet and oral hypoglycaemics and particularly if ketosis occurs, insulin therapy will be necessary, the principles of treatment being the same as in younger patients. However many old people are incapable of administering their own insulin therapy or of testing their urines, especially when vision is poor, and will require regular visits from the district nurse.

Diabetic Coma

Diabetic coma is a major feature of the disease in old age and may develop in cases hitherto judged as mild. It can occur "out of the blue" but may be precipitated by intercurrent illness, particularly infections. By no means all episodes of coma in elderly diabetics are due to diabetic coma however. Quite a proportion are due to associated stroke and some are hypoglycaemic incidents due to insulin or sulphonylureas.

Management of diabetic coma is much the same as in younger patients calling for soluble insulin and intravenous fluid replacement. Potassium depletion is common and potassium supplements are usually necessary after initial correction of dehydration. Prognosis is somewhat less good than in younger age-groups because of the greater risk of such complications as pneumonia, heart failure or vascular catastrophes.

Hyperosmolar non-ketotic diabetic coma is a variant form which is relatively frequent in the elderly and is recognised on an increasing scale. Blood sugar levels are typically very high and a high sodium is usual. Coma appears to be due to the high osmolality itself. Treatment is similar to that of the ketotic form but very large amounts of intravenous fluid may be needed to correct the extreme dehydration. Mortality is very high, major thrombotic incidents such as mesenteric infarction being a particular risk.

THYROID DISEASE IN OLD AGE

There is no clear evidence of a physiological decline of thyroid function with age. Although a decline of basal metabolic'rate can be demonstrated, this can be fully explained on the basis of the parallel decline in lean body mass. Thyroid disease however becomes more frequent in old age. Diffuse or nodular goitre and thyroid autoantibodies all become more frequent. Of greater practical relevance however is the rising frequency of thyrotoxicosis and myxoedema. We shall consider only these two conditions further.

Myxoedema has long been recognised as a fairly common disease of old age but thyrotoxicosis has been considered to be considerably less frequent. However screening of an unselected series of elderly patients admitted to a geriatric department has shown that the two diseases are both quite common, hypothyroidism occuring in 2.3% and hyperthyroidism in 1.1% (Bahemuka and Hodkinson, 1975). Many patients had not been suspected of having thyroid disease clinically so that, ideally, thyroid disease screening should be offered to all elderly patients who are admitted to hospital.

Tests of Thyroid Function

Screening for thyroid disease by simple blood tests is now possible. These rely on estimating thyroid hormones (thyroxine, T4, and tri-iodothyronine, T3) and the pituitary thyroid stimulating hormone (TSH) in the blood. Both T4 and T3 are largely bound to serum proteins, particularly to a specific carrier protein, thyroxine binding globulin. Only free hormones are physiologically active so that changes in binding capacity, for example fall in thyroxine binding globulin as a non-specific effect of illness or elevation due to cirrhosis or sex hormone therapy, complicate tests interpretation as abnormal total T4 or T3 levels may be encountered in euthyroid patients. Binding may be estimated by the T3-uptake test which allows calculation of free-thyroxine-index (FTI) and free-T3-index thus compensating for these disturbances. The most useful tests are FTI (which is low) and TSH (which is raised) in hypothyroidism whilst free-T3-index (which is raised) is most helpful in the diagnosis of thyrotoxicosis. TSH is of little value here for, though abnormally low, the relative insensitivity of the assay does not allow these values to be distinguished from low normal ones.

THYROTOXICOSIS

We have noted above that thyrotoxicosis is common but very often not recognised clinically. It is easy to overlook because the clinical picture rarely resembles the textbook descriptions of the disease. The atypical case is the rule rather than the exception in old age! An important presentation is with cardiac complications of heart failure and atrial fibrillation and such patients may have no obvious thyrotoxic stigmata. Some may fall into the category of "apathetic" thyrotoxicosis in which apathy, depression and weight loss are the principal features. Muscle weakness and fatigue are also common symptoms but may not be of much diagnostic help in the old where they are features of so many clinical conditions. Thyrotoxic eye signs are seldom prominent and it must be remembered that stare and infrequent blinking are far more commonly seen in parkinsonism or bulbar palsy.

Diagnosis thus heavily depends on either routine use of screening tests or having a high index of suspicion and performing the tests unstintingly. Radioactive iodine uptake tests are useful in confirmation of the diagnosis. Thyroid autoantibodies are often present but are of no real diagnostic value as they are quite often positive in those without thyroid disease. They do however indicate the importance of autoimmunity in the aetiology of thyroid disease as do the clinical associations of thyrotoxicosis and myxoedema with other diseases such as pernicious anaemia and diabetes in which auto-immunity is also thought to be important.

Treatment of thyrotoxicosis

Initial treatment is usually with anti-thyroid drugs of which carbimazole is the usual choice. Many cases can be managed solely by drug treatment and may remain in remission after treatment is discontinued, having been given for six months or so. However there is a fairly high likelihood of subsequent relapse. More severe cases are thus more often treated with radioactive iodine therapy which gives generally excellent results although there is a small risk of subsequent myxoedema. Surgical treatment is unusual and tends to be restricted to those with troublesome goitres or with toxic adenoma. The beta blocking agents can be used for the early symptomatic control of thyrotoxicosis until definitive treatment has had time to be effective.

MYXOEDEMA

Although many cases of myxoedema are clinically recognisable, routine screening shows that there are substantial numbers of cases that are overlooked clinically. This may be because the full clinical picture only develops after a fairly lengthy period of hypothyroidism. The clinical picture seen in old age closely resembles that in younger patients with mental and physical slowing, puffy face, croaky voice, cold intolerance, apathy and sometimes deafness, constipation or carpal tunnel syndrome. Signs of hair loss from the head or eyebrows are unreliable in old age whilst the mental changes are of greater importance and may amount to a picture of apparent dementia or more florid psychosis, often of a depressive type. "Hung-up" tendon reflexes are a very useful sign but also occur in hypothermic patients. A slow pulse is an uncommon sign in late cases. Normochromic anaemia may be seen and responds only to thyroid therapy.

Severe myxoedema is very often accompanied by ischaemic heart disease as the raised serum lipids appear to favour the rapid development of atheroma. This complication is of particular relevance in treatment as thyroid treatment may all too readily provoke acute myocardial infarction. Electrocardiography should thus be a routine requirement before treatment is started and if abnormal indicates a particularly cautious dosage regime.

Treatment of myxoedema

Treatment of myxoedema calls for life-long replacement therapy with L-thyroxine. Dosage should always be cautious but particularly where there is clinical evidence of ischaemic heart disease. It is usual to start with 0.05 mg daily and to increase this by 0.05 mg steps at fortnightly intervals. Usual maintenance doses are are around 0.15-0.2 mg per day and as thyroid is slow acting this can be given at a single occasion rather than in divided doses. TSH is a useful test to monitor dosage levels, returning to normal when adequate replacement has been given. Serum T4 may also be measured, adequate therapy usually giving mildly elevated levels.

Results of the treatment are generally good but even the most careful treatment does not entirely avoid subsequent myocardial infarction. Dementia may also prove to be irreversible, particularly when diagnosis and treatment have been delayed. It seems likely that results may be substantially better with earlier recognition of the disease such as may be achieved by the appropriate application of routine screening tests.

HYPERPARATHYROIDISM

Hyperparathyroidism due to parathyroid hyperplasia or adenoma is not rare in elderly women though it is far less common in elderly men. It is usually recognised by the finding of a consistently elevated serum calcium, the diagnosis being virtually certain when this is coupled with a normal or elevated level of serum parathormone as secretion of the hormone should be suppressed by hypercalcaemia due to other causes. It is unusual to find evidence of parathyroid bone disease in elderly women with hyperparathyroidism and only a minority have evidence of renal stone formation. The disease may be asymptomatic or may give classical symptoms of anorexia, malaise, constipation and polyuria. Progressive renal failure and progressive mental deterioration may result if the disease is left untreated so that surgical intervention is justified if the general condition of the patient permits it.

Further Reading

Exton-Smith, A N & Caird, F I (1980) Eds. Metabolic and nutritional disorders in the elderly, John Wright & Sons Ltd., Bristol.
Greenblatt, R B (1978) Ed. Geriatric endocrinology, Raven Press, New York.

21

Skeletal Disease

DISEASES OF JOINTS

Joint disease is extremely common in old age and is a major source of disability. Indeed osteoarthritic changes of some degree are virtually ubiquitous. Other chronic forms of arthritis such as rheumatoid arthritis are quite frequent and mainly represent the persistence of disease which began in middle life although they may begin in old age.

Because arthritic conditions may be considered to be almost a "normal" burden of old age, there is an obvious danger that pain or stiffness due to other diseases may be dismissed as due to "rheumatism". Thus bone pain from osteomalacia, undiagnosed fracture or malignant secondary deposits. limb pains from polyneuritis or stiffness of the limbs due to parkinsonism are examples of diseases which may be overlooked in this way. Such failures to reach the correct diagnosis are of particular importance when the overlooked disease is one for which effective treatment could have been given, for example vitamin D for osteomalacia, L dopa for parkinsonism or stilboestrol for the bone metastases of carcinoma of the prostate or breast.

Osteoarthritis

Osteoarthritis, or degenerative joint disease, is the chief form of arthritis in the elderly. Its aetiology is probably multifactorial and heredity seems to be involved as well as environmental and other factors. Obesity appears to be a factor of considerable importance for few overweight old people escape the development of significant osteoarthritis of the knees. The main pathological change in osteoarthritis is loss of articular cartilage. Joints become increasingly congruous and increased friction and crepitus result. New bone formation leads to osteophytosis as well as to sclerosis at the joint surfaces and these changes plus the loss of cartilage which results in loss of radiological "joint space" give rise to the typical radiological features.

Clinically, osteoarthritis may remain asymptomatic even when it is radiologically quite advanced but in symptomatic cases, pain, crepitus and restriction of movement are the principal manifestations. In the knee, secondary damage to ligaments may result in marked lateral instability and to eventual gross destruction which may be similar to that seen in a neuropathic joint. Osteoarthritis commonly affects multiple joints but can be asymmetrical in its distribution and commonly principally affects a particular site. Some joints tend to be spared but may develop severe osteoarthritis if subjected to abnormal stress. Thus elbows and shoulders seldom have severe osteoarthritic changes except when they have been subjected to abnormal weight bearing because of the prolonged use of walking aids such as a stick, tripod or frame.

Osteoarthritis of Hands. Osteoarthritis of the hands typically affects the thumb-base (first carpo-metacarpal joint), the 2nd and 3rd metacarpo-phalangeal joints and the terminal inter-phalangeal joints. However it is fairly common for the proximal inter-phalangeal joints to be involved also and this may lead to an incorrect diagnosis of rheumatoid arthritis being made. The sparing of the carpus in osteoarthritis and the sparing of the thumb-base in rheumatoid arthritis are useful distinguishing features of the two diseases. Although commonly giving rise to some pain, osteoarthritis of the hands seldom results in any severe disability. It is often the principal manifestation of osteoarthritis in elderly women particularly.

Osteoarthritis of Hips. Osteoarthritis of hips is less common than that of hands or knees but is particularly disabling. Fortunately it is predominantly unilateral in quite a proportion of cases. Pain may be severe and getting in and out of bed and from a chair become difficult especially when these are of low height. Flexion or adduction contractures may add considerably to the disability and the extra flexion strains put on the lumbar spine often lead to severe osteoarthritis of lumbar spine and sacro-iliac joint also.

Surgical treatment can be of immense value and may be considered even if patients are very old provided that their general condition and mental state are reasonably good. The main operations are either total hip replacement where a prosthetic acetabulum as well as femoral head is fitted or the simpler arthroplasty where only the femoral head is replaced.

Osteoarthritis of Knees. This is the form of osteoarthritis most often producing significant disability. Obesity is a frequent association and such patients may be greatly helped by successful weight reduction. Unfortunately prosthetic surgery of the knee is not yet a satisfactory procedure and is best avoided in old patients whilst arthrodesis of a severely osteoarthritic knee is usually impraticable as the resulting disability of a fixed extended leg is usually more than an elderly person can successfully cope with. Analgesics form an important part of general management but joint injection with hydrocortisone can give useful if short-lived amelioration of symptoms. Aspiration can be useful when traumatic effusion occurs and this is not an infrequent finding. Where gross lateral instability leads to great difficulty in walking light splintage of the knee with a knee corset may help to stabilise it and help both pain and mobility.

Osteoarthritis of Spine. Osteoarthritis of the spine is frequent and usually asymptomatic but may give rise to backache. Lumbar disc syndromes are extremely rare and when low back pain occurs this is often due to strain of an osteoarthritic sacro-iliac joint which may also give radiation of pain down the back of the leg. Sacro-iliac strain is recognised by marked localised tenderness over the joint and responds well to local infiltration with hydrocortisone and procaine. The possibility of malignant spinal deposits as a cause of low back pain also needs to be considered and vertebral collapse from osteoporosis is a further possibility.

Rheumatoid Arthritis

Rheumatoid arthritis only occasionally starts in old age and more usually is long-standing, having begun in middle life. In view of this many cases are "burnt out" ones with little clinical activity but often with considerable secondary degenerative joint disease. Non-articular manifestations such as Sjögren's syndrome, tendon lesions and nodules are quite often seen. Arthritis of the hands may be extreme, so called arthritis mutilans, but function in such cases may be surprisingly well maintained.

Geriatric departments tend to collect a small group of patients with rheumatoid arthritis of such a degree that they are totally incapacitated and literally do not have a single decent joint left. Such patients account for most of the minority group of long-stay patients who have normal intellect.

The treatment of rheumatoid arthritis in old age is much the same as in younger patients but as a general policy it is wise to avoid corticosteroid therapy if possible. Old patients with rheumatoid arthritis are usually severely osteoporotic in any case and steroid therapy may seriously aggravate this so that painful vertebral collapse or pathological fractures result.

Old patients with severe rheumatoid arthritis may suffer from very considerable pain but are often denied potent analgesics because of fears of the development of addiction. When likely life-span is short and pain is making existence miserable, such objections are no longer valid and potent analgesics such as pethidine or opiates should be used.

Gout

Although far less common than osteoarthritis or rheumatoid arthritis, gout is fairly common and in contrast with earlier age-groups affects women as well as men. The clinical picture remains the same as in younger patients and treatment follows the same lines. Phenylbutazone or colchicine are effective in acute attacks and long-term treatment may be with uricosuric drugs such as probenecid or with allopurinol. However long-term treatment need not always be undertaken and is probably unnecessary when there has only been an occasional acute attack especially where this was precipitated by thiazide diuretics. Treatment is indicated however where attacks have been frequent or severe or where multiple tophi have developed.

Pseudo-gout

This condition is less common than true gout but probably far more common than has been generally recognised. It gives a similar clinical picture to gout but symptoms are due to the deposition of crystals of calcium pyrophosphate and not urates as in true gout. The diagnosis can be confirmed by the demonstration of birefringent calcium pyrophosphate crystals in fluid from the affected joint and is suggested when "gout" occurs but serum uric acid is normal or where calcification of articular cartilage or of the menisci of the knee is noted radiologically. Phenylbutazone appears to be helpful in the treatment of the acute attacks.

Septic Arthritis

Pyogenic infection of isolated joints is occasionally encountered. Rheumatoid joints are particularly vulnerable but joints with only minimal osteoarthritis may be affected. The diagnosis is readily missed as elderly patients may show no severe constitutional upset but rather a non-specific deterioration. Effusions into joints of sick patients should therefore come under suspicion even though they may be painless and not giving rise to obvious inflammatory signs. Routine aspiration of such joints will avoid missing this important and treatable condition.

DISEASES OF BONE

Osteoporosis

The term osteoporosis refers to bone which is qualitatively normal but is reduced in amount, that is anatomical bone is less dense. Local osteoporosis may occur in response to various forms of disuse, bone being actively removed by osteoclastic activity. Examples are immobilisation in plaster of Paris or the hemiplegic limb where osteoporosis may be severe enough to result in pathological fracture.

Generalised osteoporosis is however a far more common and important clinical problem in the elderly, particularly in old women. Sometimes generalised osteoporosis has a clear relationship to some associated condition such as, for example, thyrotoxicosis, gastrectomy, Cushing's disease or corticosteroid therapy. More often, however, there is no such obvious explanation and it is uncertain to what extent osteoporosis is a disease, an inevitable age change, an expression of sex hormone lack or a reflection of skeletal disuse. Certainly, skeletal density reaches a peak in early adult life and undergoes a steady decline thereafter with an acceleration of bone loss in females after the menopause.

Osteoporosis is totally asymptomatic until a degree of structural weakness occurs which leads to mechanical failure of the bone in the form of fracture or collapse. Either may occur pathologically or as a result of some degree of trauma. There is no biochemical disturbance except that alkaline phosphatase may rise after fracture or collapse for some time. The high incidences of fracture of the femur, humerus and of Colles' fracture in old age are largely attributable to the high prevalence of osteoporosis. Vertebral collapse is common and may occur acutely, especially when trauma is involved, and give severe back pain. More often collapsed vertebra are found incidentally and appear never to have given significant pain. It may be that vertebral collapse has occured as a gradual process in these patients. Vertebral collapse is a major cause of kyphosis and may also be recognised by the presence of a keratinised transverse abdominal skin crease, by the occurrence of apposition of the lower ribs and pelvic brim and by the loss of trunk height.

Treatment with anabolic steroids, calcium supplements and other regimes have their protagonists but are not of proven value and are not advised in the elderly patient. Sex hormone replacement therapy in postmenopausal women has been shown to arrest bone loss. Unfortunately, accelerated bone loss supervenes if the treatment is discontinued later. The patient may then finish up with more bone loss than if she had never been treated. In view of this, replacement therapy implies a commitment to life-long maintenance of treatment which is of dubious practicality and safety.

Osteomalacia

Osteomalacia is a generalised disease of bone in which osteoid matrix is formed normally but then fails to undergo proper calcification. An excess of uncalcified osteoid accumulates and the bone becomes softer. Osteomalacia is of considerable importance in the elderly because it is reasonably common (Anderson and his colleagues (1966) reporting a 4 per cent incidence in female admissions to a geriatric department), and gives rise to serious morbidity and yet is eminently treatable once recognised. However the clinical picture can be an unobtrusive or misleading one so that the diagnosis needs to be actively sought for, there being a good case for routine biochemical screening of patients at risk, particularly housebound elderly women. Bone pain is the most specific manifestation but can all too readily be ascribed to arthritis or other causes. Muscle weakness may be a striking feature and affects particularly the proximal groups and may give a typical waddling gait. Fractures may occur, particularly of ribs but sometimes of femur.

The typical biochemical changes are that serum calcium is either abnormally low or in the low normal range, serum phosphate is low and alkaline phosphatase is raised. Unfortunately not all cases show all these changes and many other conditions can produce them individually so that biochemical changes usually suggest rather than prove the diagnosis. Radiology may be diagnostic if Looser's zones are present (pseudo-fractures); these are bands of decalcification more or less at right angles to the surface of the bone and are most often seen in the femur, ribs, pubis or scapula. Otherwise proof of the diagnosis depends on the demonstration of an excess of osteoid on the trabecular surfaces of bone examined as undecalcified sections. Bone biopsy can be readily obtained by trephine biopsy of the iliac crest using local anaesthesia.

Osteomalacia due to Vitamin D lack. Most cases of osteomalacia can be attributed to vitamin D lack or to its malabsorption. Vitamin D is supplied both by the diet and by synthesis on the skin surface for which ultra-violet light exposure is needed. Simple deficiency may thus occur in housebound old people who must rely entirely on their dietary intake and this is often low in old age. The risk is greater when the patient has been housebound for a long time for even minor exposure to sun or even to bright daylight out of doors seems to be sufficient to allow skin synthesis. In rather more old people malabsorption is an additional factor and post-gastrectomy syndrome in old women provides the largest group of moderate and severe osteomalacia cases in geriatric practice.

Drug-induced Osteomalacia. Barbiturates and some other drugs which lead to enzyme induction in the liver may result in osteomalacia and this most often occurs as a complication of the treatment of epilepsy. The liver normally converts vitamin D to a more active metabolite 25 hydroxy-cholecalciferol but in situations of enzyme induction it appears that this in turn suffers rapid metabolism to inactive compounds.

Osteomalacia in Immigrants. Osteomalacia is much more common in immigrants from the Indian sub-continent than in the native population. As elderly immigrants are no longer a rarity this has relevance to geriatric practice although the observations extend to all age-groups. It has been suggested that it is the high phytate content of the traditional diet of such immigrants which may account for their vulnerability. Phytate occurs in the roughage of cereals but is partially destroyed during the leavening process of baking. The unleavened chapatti provides a phytate intake which may be sufficient to seriously interfere with calcium absorption from the gut by the formation of complexes and so lead to a higher vitamin D requirement and thus osteomalacia. However others have questioned this explanation and believe that dietary lack and poor sunlight exposure alone can explain the observed high incidences of the disease.

Osteomalacia in Renal Failure. A proportion of cases of osteomalacia occur in renal failure. A different mechanism may be responsible here. After conversion to 25 hydroxy-cholecalciferol by the liver it appears that this in turn is changed to a far more active substance, 1,25 dihydroxy-cholecalciferol, which is believed to be the substance actually involved in the control of calcium absorption from the gut. It seems likely that in renal failure this conversion is less able to be effected so that vitamin D has less biological effectiveness and unless available in large amounts osteomalacia results.

Treatment of Osteomalacia. Treatment of osteomalacia is one of the more satisfying therapeutic activities in geriatrics. Response to vitamin D is sometimes little short of miraculous, an irritable, uncooperative and helpless patient being transformed within a few days into an active, cheerful and pain free individual.

Where osteomalacia is due to simple vitamin lack only small doses of vitamin D may be necessary and it is then convenient to use tabs. calcium and vitamin D (B.P.) which provide 500 i.u. of vitamin D per tablet. However where there is malabsorption and in renal failure where there is resistance to vitamin D therapy, large doses tend to be necessary and calciferol tablets (1.25 mg) which each provide 50,000 i.u. are more suitable. In more severe cases it is possibly advantageous to give calcium supplements in addition to vitamin D.

Biochemical monitoring of treatment is essential for dosage has to be regulated by trial and error using serum calcium as the guide. Over-treatment can lead to dangerous hypercalcaemia so monitoring may need to be frequent initially. Calcium and phosphate respond quickly to treatment but alkaline often rises at first and then may take some months to return completely to normal. Most patients will need a permanent maintenance dose of vitamin D but some patients with simple vitamin lack can stop treatment after a few months provided that they avoid future relapse by attention to their diet and sunlight exposure.

Paget's Disease

This is a localised and patchy bone disease of unknown aetiology, the incidence of which rises with age. It is found in something like five percent of geriatric patients. The bones most often involved are pelvis, lumbar spine, femora, tibiae, clavicles, skull and humeri but any bone may be involved. Bones become expanded and softer and may become deformed, for example the characteristic bowing of femora or tibiae. Histologically Paget's disease is characterised by abnormally active but chaotic remodelling. Radiologically it may appear denser but normal fine architecture is distorted and the bones are mechanically weak so that fracture is an important complication. Limb bones may show typical transverse fractures. Affected bones are also far more vascular and when Paget's disease is particularly extensive this may lead to high output cardiac failure or may facilitate the development of hypothermia due to increased heat loss. An uncommon but important manifestation is bone pain consisting of boring or throbbing pain over the involved bones. Other complications are those due to the enlargement of the bones which may result in foraminal encroachment of which deafness is the most important example. The most serious complication is the development of bone sarcoma in an affected bone. The frequency of this was undoubtedly overstated in the older literature and more recent work has indicated that sarcoma may arise in as little as 0.2 per cent of cases. However the vast majority of cases are totally asymptomatic and only come to light as an incidental finding on X-ray or because of the finding of a high alkaline phosphatase, a common accompaniment of the disease.

Treatment is therefore only needed in a small proportion of cases. Fracture calls for standard orthopaedic management and Pagetic bone heals at a normal rate. Sarcoma carries a very poor prognosis and may require amputation or radiotherapy. Medical treatment is indicated in only two situations, bone pain that does not respond to simple analgesics and which is definitely from the involved bone itself and not from arthritis of the adjacent joint and high output failure due to extensive disease. The drug of choice is calcitonin, a hormone with a hypocalcaemic action which is secreted by the thyroid. This has to be given by daily injection either in the form of the porcine or synthetic human hormone and results in striking relief of pain and reduction of bone turnover and vascularity. Alternative treatments are the antibiotic mithramycin or the hormone glucagon, both of which may act by stimulating endogenous calcitonin release, or the use of diphosphonates such as disodium etidronate. This last appears to inhibit new bone formation by acting as a crystal poison. These alterantive treatments are to be regarded as essentially experimental at the present time. Even calcitonin therapy, although of undoubted short term benefit in carefully selected cases, remains to be fully evaluated, particularly in regard to the effects of its long term use.

22

Diseases of the Blood and Reticulo-endothelial System

ANAEMIA

Anaemia is common in ill old people and indeed is not rare in apparently healthy old people in the community. However the haematological criteria of normality are not significantly different in old age, such haematological age changes that have been demonstrated being of little practical significance with the possible exception of the lower range for the white cell count. Minor changes are for red cell size to increase very slightly with age and for the upper limit of normal of the E.S.R. to rise, probably as a consequence of age trends for albumin and globulin, which tend to show a fall and a rise with age respectively.

Anaemia, usually taken to be a haemoglobin concentration of less than 12 G/100ml, manifests itself in old age much as in youth. However the vague and slowly progressive symptoms of anaemia in an old person run a higher risk of being ignored or of being ascribed to old age itself. Important manifestations in the old are palpitation, breathlessness, postural hypotension, giddiness and the onset of congestive cardiac failure or of left ventricular failure. Confusional states are not particularly associated with anaemia in general but are an important part of the clinical picture of pernicious anaemia.

Investigation of anaemia in old age should follow the same lines as in the young and will not be detailed here. The temptation to omit proper investigation and to treat clinically diagnosed anaemia with blunderbuss therapy of iron and B_{12} and folate should be strongly resisted.

Iron Deficiency Anaemia

Iron deficiency anaemia is by far the most important category. Although poor dietary intake of iron may often be a contributory factor, pure dietary iron deficiency would take many years to develop because of the efficiency of the normal conservation mechanisms and must be a considerable rarity. Abnormal iron loss virtually always plays a part and is most often from the gastrointestinal tract. Hiatus hernia heads the list but peptic ulcer, diverticular disease, piles and cancers of the gastrointestinal tract must all be considered. Drugs producing gastric bleeding may also be important and aspirin and phenylbutazone are the most important of these. Blood loss from the gut is so often a factor that testing for occult blood in the faeces should be mandatory in any unexplained case of iron deficiency anaemia.

Treatment is normally with oral iron, ferrous sulphate being cheap and effective, but when poorly tolerated or if the patient cannot be relied upon to take the pills, intramuscular iron-dextran (imferon) is the best alternative.

Sometimes apparently iron deficient anaemia, that is hypochromic microcytic anaemia, may occur which does not respond to iron therapy and indeed investigation may show normal iron stores. Such "sideroblastic" anaemia may occur in association with chronic diseases but some respond to treatment with pyridoxine.

The Megaloblastic Anaemias

Modern automated haematological techniques such as provided by the "Coulter S" machine allow very accurate determination of red cell size and have shown that macrocytosis is quite common in ill old people, even when they have no anaemia. This may be due to quite a variety of causes.

Pernicious Anaemia. Pernicious anaemia is the most important cause of macrocytosis in old age. The Coulter S now often leads to its recognition in a pre-anaemic stage because the increase in cell size is the earlier change and thus pre-symptomatic treatment is made possible. Pernicious anaemia is due to vitamin B_{12} deficiency due to an impairment of its absorption which is secondary to lack of Intrinsic Factor. This is a factor which assists absorption and is secreted by gastric parietal cells. It is thought that the failure of intrinsic factor production in pernicious anaemia is due to autoimmune phenomena which also produce the accompanying achlorhydria and underlie the associations with other autoimmune conditions such as thyrotoxicosis, myxoedema, diabetes and rheumatoid arthritis.

In addition to true pernicious anaemia, similar megaloblastic anaemia due to B_{12} deficiency can occur as a result of loss of parietal cell area as a result of gastrectomy or to malabsorption of the vitamin due to small bowel disease or its excessive loss by sequestration in blind loop syndromes or small bowel diverticula.

Pernicious anaemia has an insidious onset but may progress to a stage of very severe anaemia, when slight associated icterus is common. A smooth atrophic tongue is a characteristic but by no means invariable feature. Anorexia and vague dyspepsia may occur and patients may lose a considerable amount of weight. Mental confusion may be marked so that severe dementia may sometimes be simulated. An occasional but grave complication which may occur before there is any significant anaemia is subacute combined degeneration of the cord. The cord signs are pyramidal signs and evidence of position sense and vibration sense loss and are usually accompanied by signs of a mild peripheral neuropathy. With prompt treatment this is completely reversible but delay in diagnosis and treatment may result in permanent damage.

Diagnosis of pernicious anaemia is confirmed by the finding of a megalo-blastic marrow coupled with a low serum B_{12} level and evidence of mal-absorption of the vitamin which is improved by administration of intrinsic factor (Schilling test). It is not usually necessary to confirm the presence of achlorhydria and old patients should generally be spared the unpleasantness of intubation for this purpose.

Treatment of Pernicious Anaemia. Treatment is to give B_{12} by injection and to continue this regularly for life. The vitamin is more effective in the form of hydroxy-cobalamin and may be given in doses of 1000 μG twice weekly until a good haematological response has been achieved and monthly thereafter. Subacute combined degeneration of the cord calls for more frequent administration, daily or alternate days, until full response occurs. It is vital not to give folate as this exacerbates the neurological damage. For this reason folate should never be given in megaloblastic anaemia without proper investigation.

Folate Deficiency. Folate deficiency is far less often the cause of macrocytosis than is B_{12} deficiency but is none the less fairly often seen in ill old people. Body stores can be fairly rapidly depleted so that marginal folate deficiency can develop in ill people who are eating poorly. However this rarely produces actual megaloblastic anaemia, clinical cases of which most commonly have some type of malabsorption syndrome as their underlying cause.

Other Causes of Macrocytosis. Quite a number of instances of macrocytosis may be encountered in elderly patients who do not have megaloblastic anaemia. The most frequent example is macrocytosis due to alcohol and this can be a useful pointer to the possibility that a patient's problems are due to alcoholism. Myxoedema may also give macrocytosis whilst less frequent causes include aplastic anaemia, cirrhosis, carcinoma and reticulosis.

Normocytic Anaemias

Anaemia without change in cell size may occur after haemorrhage or in haemolytic or hypoplastic anaemias but more commonly in old age may be seen in association with chronic diseases. These "symptomatic" anaemias are of obscure cause and do not respond to treatment with haematinics.

Anaemia of Infection. Normochromic normocytic anaemia may be seen in a variety of chronic infections such as chronic sepsis with sinus or abscess formation, large pressure sores or chronic pyelonephritis. Such anaemia may be an important pointer to more obscure types of infection such as miliary tuberculosis, subacute bacterial endocarditis or occult sepsis such as an unrecognised empyema or pyonephrosis.

Anaemia of Chronic Disease. Symptomatic anaemias also occur in other chronic diseases apart from those due to infection. The anaemia of chronic renal failure and of rheumatoid arthritis are frequent and important examples. Malignant disease is another major cause. Normochromic normo-cytic anaemia may occur with carcinoma or in reticuloses and in some instances immature red and white cell precursors appear in the peripheral blood, the so called "leucoerythroblastic" blood picture which can be an important pointer to the diagnosis of neoplastic illness.

MYELOPROLIFERATIVE DISORDERS

The Leukaemias

The Leukaemias are not rare in old age. Acute forms, particularly myelo-monocytic leukaemia, are seen occasionally and carry a bad prognosis. The most common form is chronic lymphatic leukaemia which is compatible with a survival of many years and which may remain practically asymptomatic for very long periods. It may give very high white counts and lead to some degree of normocytic anaemia and moderate lymphadenopathy is usual. Less commonly there is splenomegaly also. In some cases thrombocytopenia develops and may give rise to purpura or to more serious haemorrhagic manifestations. Treatment is often unnecessary but when indicated, cytotoxic agents such as chlorambucil may be used with benefit.

Myeloma

Myeloma has its peak incidence in old age. It is most often seen in the form of multiple myelomatosis, that is abnormal proliferation of plasma cells with foci scattered through the marrow. The condition may be asymptomatic for years and only brought to light by the finding of a very high E.S.R. during investigation for other reasons. Symptomatic cases may present with general malaise, weight loss, anaemia or with pain or patho-logical fracture due to lytic bone deposits. Some patients suffer from repeated episodes of infection and others may develop chronic renal failure. Apart from the very high E.S.R., the finding of a paraprotein band on serum protein electrophoresis, excess of plasma cells on marrow examination and Bence-Jones proteinuria are the main diagnostic aids.

Prognosis of myeloma once the symptomatic stage is reached is generally poor, particularly once renal failure occurs. Cytotoxic drugs such as melphalan or cyclophosphamide probably have little effect on overall survival time but may give dramatic tumour shrinkage and useful symptomatic relief. Severely anaemic patients may need blood transfusion. It is very doubtful that treatment of the asymptomatic case confers any benefit.

Polycythaemia

The polycythaemias are conditions characterised by an increase in the red cell mass which can be measured using chromium labelled red cells. The possibility of polycythaemia is raised by the finding of an abnormally high haemoglobin or haematocrit value though, in elderly patients, these findings are more often due to conditions in which plasma volume is decreased rather than red cell mass increased.

When a true polycythaemia is found it may be secondary to such causes as chronic respiratory failure or due to polycythaemia rubra vera. In this disease there is usually an increase in white cells and platelets as well as of red cells. The haematocrit may be very high indeed and blood viscosity is greatly increased. This favours thrombosis and the most common presentation of polycythaemia rubra vera in old age is with cerebral thrombosis. Diagnosis can be confirmed by the demonstration of an increased red cell mass using chromium labelled red cells. Treatment may be by regular venesection or more permanent control may be obtained by using radioactive phosphorus given intravenously.

Tumours of Lymphoid Tissue

Reticuloses such as lymphosarcoma, reticulum cell sarcoma and Hodgkin's disease are all encountered from time to time in old age. Their general features and treatment are similar to those in middle life.

The presence of lymphadenopathy is unusual in old age and strongly points to the possibility of one of these diseases or to chronic lymphatic leukaemia.

23

The Challenge of Geriatrics

THE DEVELOPMENT OF GERIATRICS

Geriatrics is a young specialty which is still actively growing and developing. The numbers of old people in the community continue to rise so that geriatrics will have to expand substantially, particularly if standards are to rise. Geriatrics will thus need to attract an increasing number of people to its ranks and these will include nurses, rehabilitation personnel and social workers as well as doctors.

Geriatrics has achieved spectacular growth during the first third of a century of its effective existence in Britain, the number of consultants in the specialty, for example, having roughly doubled each decade. Yet this growth has never been easy and the recruitment of doctors, nurses and paramedical workers of suitable calibre has always been difficult and remains so today. Why should this be so? Work with the elderly is less obviously rewarding than that with the young and furthermore it has been accorded lower status and prestige, most especially by doctors themselves. Added to this the physical resources provided for geriatrics were generally poor, sometimes scandalously bad, whilst elderly patients suffered from the poor esteem for age and fears of growing old and dying which were common attitudes of younger age-groups. Treatment of the elderly tended to be regarded as ineffective and a waste of time and the care of the elderly as an irksome burden on the community in general and the health professions in particular.

Geriatrics has had to work hard to modify such attitudes and has had considerable successes. More enlightened views are now far more general and the public and government are fully aware of the need for major improvements in our provision for the elderly. The Health Advisory Service has played an important part in this shaping of official attitudes. Professional attitudes have also moved forwards as is shown, for example, by such key publications as the "Report of the Working Party on Medical Care of the Elderly" (Royal College of Physicians, 1977). However a vocal if small professional opposition persists (for example, Leonard, 1976) defending obsolescent negative attitudes which were once predominant.

Teaching of geriatric medicine and work with the elderly are now integral parts of the training of medical students, nurses and therapists whilst new Chairs of geriatric medicine have been established in more than a dozen medical schools within the last decade. This exposure is valuable though perhaps less crucial than work with the elderly after qualification. What might be termed "accidental" exposure to geriatric work is how most geriatricians, myself included, seem to have first come into the specialty. For many years University College Hospital was the only English medical school with its own geriatric department. It is surely no coincidence that over those years it provided a giant's share of graduates who became geriatricians.

ADVANTAGES OF GERIATRICS

Personal exposure to geriatric work effectively demonstrates the many advantages of geriatrics to those who are sufficiently able to remove the blindfold of prejudice. Perhaps the most important attribute of geriatrics is that it is a truly general subject, paediatrics among hospital specialties being its only real rival in this respect. It embraces the whole of general medicine of the elderly but in addition rehabilitation, psychiatry of old age, sociology and gerontology are important and interesting additions. Furthermore the running of a geriatric department gives an opportunity for the development and deployment of administrative, managerial and medico-political skills. It is a profoundly satisfying specialty for the person with all-round abilities with an appeal that is quite opposite from that of the narrow "super-specialties" into which present day medicine is tending to become increasingly fragmented. Geriatrics is clearly concerned with the whole patient and indeed with the whole of the elderly population of the local catchment area. It imposes a salutary discipline of "the buck stops here".

Elderly patients, although they might seem at superficial consideration to be rather unprepossessing, are a pleasure to work with. They have seen doctors come and doctors go during their long lives and are not too easy to over-impress nor easily over-awed. They have a down to earth, often earthily humourous and essentially philosophical attitude to doctors and to illness. This and the very nature of geriatric work and its clear therapeutic limitations ensure that the geriatrician assumes no role of remote and godlike infallibility, a part some groups of patients seem to wish upon their doctors but surely neither a comfortable nor useful one to accept. One is sometimes asked if the frequency of death in geriatric work does not make it very depressing for the doctor. It is not, for the geriatrician has not adopted the role of infallibility and so does not have to regard his patient's death as a humiliating failure. More important are the attitudes of the elderly patients themselves. We can learn much from them by observing their mature approach to death and illness and the more we see of the elderly, the greater our respect for them.

The "pioneer" aspects of geriatrics are an added attraction. Nothing in geriatrics is cut and dried, departments run on very different lines from each other and each geriatrician can feel free to follow his own inclinations and explore new approaches to his work. It is far easier for the geriatrician to be able to make a difference to the character and quality of a local service. Indeed the basic organisational techniques of geriatrics are still being actively developed and every geriatrician is capable of making a meaningful contribution. This applies with equal force to research in the geriatric field. Geriatricians have only just begun to open up the enormous research potential of their subject and unrivalled opportunities lie ahead. It needs no exceptional qualities or genius to be able to make useful contributions to the expanding fields of clinical, biochemical, clinico-pathological, socio-medical, psychogeriatric, organisational or experimental research in geriatrics. Furthermore much useful research can be done without the need for expensive equipment of facilities. An enquiring mind and some persistence are all that is necessary.

GERIATRICS AS A CAREER

Apart from the appeal of geriatric work itself, there are sound practical reasons for choosing to make a career in this specialty. Geriatrics is clearly destined to continue to expand for many years to come, both to catch up with present under-provision and to keep pace with the increasing size of the age-group. Clearly it is a specialty which is not at any risk of a future eclipse such as the fields of chest medicine or infectious diseases have already experienced! Geriatrics is at present a "four star" specialty, that is one which is officially recognised as providing exceptionally good career prospects to the new entrant and it seems virtually certain that this will continue to be so for many years to come. Promotion to consultant level is unimpeded because there is no artificial hold-up once a senior registrar has an adequate training. The trained senior registrar is not merely assured of a consultant post but is well able to choose which post in what is essentially a seller's market. Established consultants can often move to a post which they find more attractive, a freedom which is rare in other specialties.

Not only have consultant posts increased in number but there have been improvements in their quality. The size of departments has been brought down over the years or further posts have been created in large ones. Physical resources tend to be far better than in the past and are improving perhaps more rapidly than in any other field, although there is a lot of room for improvement in many instances. The Department has now accepted the principle that geriatric departments ought to have admission beds in the district general hospital, ensuring that the professional isolation resulting from the practice of geriatrics in separate geriatric hospitals will be brought to an end. There are also an increasing number of teaching hospital and academic posts in geriatric medicine which are helping the further integration of the specialty into the mainstream of hospital medicine and also provide improving career prospects.

Geriatric medicine has a special appeal to those whose approach to medicine is broadly based rather than narrowly specialised. The young doctor entering this branch of medicine can be confident that it has a very wide breadth of interest and that its career prospects are difficult to match. Furthermore the young doctor will be investing his future in a field which really needs his skills and commitment and which has great social importance. Geriatrics is indeed the greatest challenge within medicine today.

References

Adams, G. F. (1971). Clinical outlook for stroke patients. *Gerontologia clinica* **13**, 181-188.
Anderson, I., Campbell, A. E. R., Dunn, A. and Runciman, J. B. M. (1966). Osteomalacia in elderly women. *Scottish med. J.* **2**, 420-435.
Asher, R. A. J. (1947). The dangers of bed. *Brit, med J.* **2**, 967-968.
Bahemuka, M. and Hodkinson, H. M. (1975). Screening for hypothyroidism in elderly inpatients. *Brit. med J.* **2**, 601-603.
Bedford, P. D. and Caird, F. I. (1960). Valvular Disease of the Heart in Old Age. Churchill, London.
Bowen, D. M. and Davison, A. N. (1978). Biochemical changes in normal ageing of the brain and in dementia. *In* "Recent Advances in Geriatric Medicine" (Ed. B. Isaacs), p. 41-59. Churchill Livingstone, Edinburgh.
Brocklehurst, J. C. and Shergold, M. (1968). What happens when geriatric patients leave hospital? *Lancet* **2**, 1133-1135.
Brown, A. D. G. (1978). Gynaecological disorders in the elderly. *In* "Textbook of Geriatric Medicine and Gerontology" (Ed. J. C. Brocklehurst), p. 326-337. Churchill Livingstone, Edinburgh.
Burkitt, D. P. (1971). Possible Relationships Between Bowel Cancer and Dietary Habits. *Proc. roy. Soc. Med.* **64**, 964-965.
Coleman, J. A. and Denham, M. J. (1980). Perforation of peptic ulceration in the elderly. *Age Ageing* **9**, 257-261.
Dall, J. L. C. (1970). Maintenance digoxin in elderly patients. *Brit. med. J.* **2**, 705-706.
Davies, M. J. (1971). Pathology of the Conducting Tissue of the Heart. Butterworth, London.
Dayan, A. D. (1978) Neuropathology of aging. *In* "Textbook of Geriatric Medicine and Gerontology" (Ed. J. C. Brocklehurst), 2nd Edn, p. 158-184. Churchill Livingstone, Edinburgh.
Denham, M. J., Farran, H. and James, G. (1973). The value of ^{125}I fibrinogen in the diagnosis of deep vein thrombosis in hemiplegia. *Age Ageing* **2**, 207-210.
Denham, M. J., Hodkinson, H. M. and Fisher, M. (1975) Glomerular filtration rate in sick elderly patients. *Age Ageing* **4**, 32-36.
Department of Health and Social Security (1970). First Report by the Panel on Nutrition of the Elderly. *Rep. Publ. Hlth. Med.* Sub. no. 123, H.M.S.O., London.
Department of Health and Social Security (1972). Nutrition Survey of the Elderly. *Rep. Publ. Hlth. Med.* Sub. no. 3, H.M.S.O., London.
Durnin, J. V. G. A. (1978). Nutrition. *In* "Textbook of Geriatric Medicine and Gerontology" (Ed. J. C. Brocklehurst), 2nd Edn, p. 417-432. Churchill Livingstone. Edinburgh.
Exton-Smith, A. N. (1978). Disturbances of autonomic regulation. *In* "Recent Advances in Geriatric Medicine" (Ed. B. Isaacs), p. 85-100. Churchill Livingstone, Edinburgh.
Hall, M. R. P. (1973). The assessment of the value of three types of hearing aid to overcome the communication barrier of deafness in the elderly patient in the hospital setting. *Age Ageing* **2**, 125-127.
Hayward, G. W. (1973). Ineffective Endocarditis: A Changing Disease—1. *Brit. med. J.* **2**, 706-709.
Hodkinson, H. M. (1972). Evaluation of a mental test score for assessment of mental impairment in the elderly. *Age Ageing* **1**, 233-237.
Hodkinson, H. M. (1972). More favourable prognosis of motor neurone disease in old age. *Age Ageing* **1**, 182-184.
Hodkinson, H. M. (1973). Mental impairment in the elderly. *J. roy. Coll. Physns.* **7**, 305-317.

Hodkinson, H. M. (1977). Biochemical diagnosis of the elderly. Chapman and Hall, London.
Hodkinson, H. M. and Hodkinson, I. (1980). Death and discharge from a geriatric department. *Age Ageing* **9**, 220-228.
Hodkinson, H. M. and Jefferys, P. M. (1972). Making hospital geriatrics work. *Brit. med. J.* **4**, 536-539.
Hodkinson, H. M. and Pomerance, A. (1979). The clinical pathology of heart failure and atrial fibrillation in old age. *Postgrad. med. J.* **55**, 251-254.
Isaacs, B. (1971). Geriatric patients—do their families care? *Brit. med. J.* **4**, 282-286.
Keating, F. R., Jones, J. D., Elveback, L. R. and Randall, R. V. (1969). The relation of age and sex to the distribution of values in healthy adults of serum calcium, inorganic phosphorus, magnesium, alkaline phosphatase, total proteins, albumin and blood urea. *J. Lab. clin. med.* **73**, 825-838.
Lancet Editorial (1971). Care of the Dying. *Lancet* **2**, 753-754.
Leask, R. G. S., Andrews, G. R. and Caird, F. I. (1973). Normal values of sixteen blood constituents in the elderly. *Age Ageing* **2**, 14-23.
Leonard, J. C. (1976). Can geriatrics survive? *Brit. med. J.* **1**, 1335-1336.
McKeown, T. (1960). *In* "Ageing, its Changes and its Promise", p. 55-61. National Old People's Welfare Council, London.
Moore-Smith, B. (1980). The management of hypertension in the elderly. *In* "The Treatment of Medical Problems in the Elderly" (Ed. M. J. Denham), p. 117-158. MTP Press, Lancaster.
Post, F. (1978). Psychiatric disorders. *In* "Textbook of Geriatric Medicine and Gerontology" (Ed. J. C. Brocklehurst), 2nd Edn, p. 185-200. Churchill, Livingstone, Edinburgh.
Prakash, C. and Stern, G. (1973). Neurological signs in the elderly. *Age Ageing* **2**, 24-27.
Pulvertaft, C. N. (1972). Experiences with peptic ulcer in elderly men in York. *Age Ageing* **1**, 24-29.
Roberts, L. B. (1967). The normal ranges with statistical analysis for seventeen blood constituents. *Clin. chim. acta.* **16**, 69-78.
Rosin, A. J. and Boyd, R. V. (1966). Complications of illness in geriatric hospital patients. *J. Chron. Dis.* **19**, 307-313.
Royal College of Physicians of London (1966). Report of the Committee on Accidental Hypothermia. Royal College of Physicians, London.
Royal College of Physicians of London (1977). Report of the working party on medical care of the elderly. Royal College of Physicians, London.
Saunders, C. (1971). A Death in the Family: A Professional View. *Brit. med. J.* **1**, 30-31.
Sourander, L. B. (1978). The aging kidney. *In* "Textbook of Geriatric Medicine and Gerontology" (Ed. J. C. Brocklehurst), p. 291-305. Churchill Livingstone, Edinburgh.
Townsend, P. (1962). The last refuge. Routledge and Kegan Paul, London.
Walton, K. W. (1978). Atherosclerosis and aging. *In* "Textbook of Geriatric Medicine and Gerontology" (Ed. J. C. Brocklehurst), 2nd Edn, p. 89-116. Churchill Livingstone, Edinburgh.
Wartenberg, R. (1952). Head-dropping test. *Brit. med. J.* **1**, 687-689.

INDEX

Stair climbing, 48
Statistics concerning the elderly, 31
Stilboestrol, 29
Stokes-Adams attacks, 30, 99
Stomach carcinoma, 114-5
Streptococcus viridans infection, 100
Stricture formation, 112
Stroke, 119-24
Subdural haematoma, 28, 124
Sulphonylurea oral drugs, unnecessary treatment, 75
Support, social, need for, 8
Symptoms, missing, 27
Systemic arterial embolism, 110-1

T

T3 and T4, 23, 138-9
Tachycardia, 98
Temperature responses, altered, 27
Tendon reflexes, 17
Terminal care, 65-9
Therapeutic environment, 43-5
Thiamine, 76
Thrombo-embolic disease, 109-11
Thrombo-embolism, 24, 29, 109-11
Thrombosis, venous, 29, 109
Thyroid
    disease, 23, 138-40
    function tests, 22-3, 138-9
Thyrotoxicosis, 139
Thyroxine, 22, 140
Thyroxine-binding globulin, 22
Tietze's syndrome, 96
Tongue, dry, 16

Tuberculosis,
    miliary, 93, 152
    pulmonary, 21, 93
Tumour, brain, 28, 124-5
Turgor assessment, 15

U

Ulcers, rodent, 19
Uraemia, 29, 83, 130-2
Urea levels, 22, 23
Uric acid, 22, 23
Urinalysis, 24
Urinary infection, 24, 83, 132-5
Urinary retention, 18
Uro-genital system,
    diseases, 130-5
    examination, 18

V

Valvular disease of heart, 96-8
Venous thrombosis, 29, 109
Vertebral collapse, 18, 145-6
    painless, 26
Vitamin B_{12}
    deficiency, 28, 84, 151-2
    requirements, 76
Vitamin D requirements, 76, 147
Vitamin deficiency, 78
Voluntary homes, 37

W

Walking, retraining, 50-2
Warden flatlets, 33-4
Warts, senile, 19
Welfare Homes, 36-7
White cell count, 22